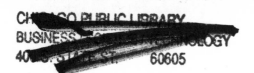

D1219145

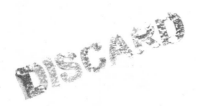

High velocity missile wounds

M. S. Owen-Smith OStJ, MS, FRCS, FRCSEd

Joint Professor of Military Surgery, Royal Army
Medical College and Royal College of Surgeons of
England; lately Hunterian Professor, Royal College
of Surgeons of England

with a Foreword by
Lord Smith of Marlow, KBE, MS, FRCS

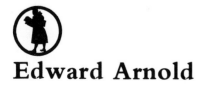

Edward Arnold

© M. S. Owen-Smith, 1981.

First published 1981
by Edward Arnold (Publishers) Ltd.
41 Bedford Square, London WC1B 3DQ

British Library Cataloguing in Publication Data
Owen-Smith, M S
  High velocity missile wounds.
  1. Gunshot wounds
  I. Title
  617'.145   RD96.3
  ISBN 0-7131-4371-1

Set in Monophoto 11/12 pt Bembo and printed in Great Britain by
Butler & Tanner Ltd, Frome and London

Foreword

by Lord Smith of Marlow

A book about wounds caused by bullets and explosives in peace time? Well, why not?

In fact there are several reasons why this particular book is most timely. To start with, it is remarkable how quickly the lessons learnt in time of war are forgotten as soon as hostilities cease. Surgeons in World War II, anxious to record for the use of others the lessons painfully wrung from bitter experience in the treatment of battle casualties, all too often, as they consulted the literature from earlier days, found that they had merely been retracing the steps trodden by their predecessors in World War I. The dangers of primary suture of wounds, the principles of surgical debridement, secondary suture and so on, were all subjects debated in surgical journals in one war, then forgotten, to be rediscovered in the next and examined as if they were new topics debated for the first time. It is good that an authoritative work shall try and introduce an element of continuity into this important branch of surgery.

A second reason is that the last few decades have seen a horrifying increase in violence involving guns and explosives and of terrorism among civilian populations, so that 'peace time' is perhaps an inaccurate description of the situation in which society now exists.

Today, any surgeon in any hospital in any city in the world may suddenly be called upon to treat a patient with a gunshot wound, or several patients injured by the explosion of a bomb, whilst the organization of any hospital may, without warning, be tested by the sudden need to receive a large number of casualties from a major terrorist outrage.

The information in this book is very complete and arranged in a logical sequence. As a preliminary to consideration of clinical aspects, a most useful section upon the mechanism of injury provides a much needed basis of understanding of the physical effects upon living tissues of both bullet wounds and injuries by explosives. The management of the injured patient and the treatment of the injuries themselves are then considered, both generally and regionally, with a final short, but informative, chapter on body armour.

iii

Despite its completeness, this is not a long book, its style being attractively concise. For this reason, although it will undoubtedly become the reference book to which many will automatically turn, it is also a book which ought to be read by all surgeons and all those in training to become surgeons. This, in fact, is no hardship for it is a most readable book and one can enjoy it and profit from it at one and the same time.

Preface

The wounds from high velocity bullets and fragments from explosive devices have always been a major feature of the many wars that have occurred in various parts of the world. They seem an inescapable fact of life, reflecting upon the failure of men to live in peaceful harmony together, regrettably these wounds which had hitherto been known as 'war wounds' now occur in all parts of the world other than in wartime. They occur because there are large numbers of the weapons of war available for the use of any faction or group that decides to attempt to settle its differences with other groups by force of arms. This means that we must now be prepared to receive and treat such wounds in all hospitals. To do this we must understand how bullets and explosive blast create wounds, study the physical phenomena concerned and from this scientific study understand the pathology of the wounds that have been created. We must know the principles of treatment based upon the pathology and finally, deal with specific treatment for the various organs and systems of the body that have been damaged. These principles have been well laid down in the past but unfortunately there has been little communication between those who know how to manage these wounds, particularly after times of war, and those who are totally ignorant of the unusual mechanisms of injury and the special techniques of management of high velocity wounds. This means that when a young surgeon meets such a wound for the first time he is likely to treat it by conventional surgical methods with disaster for the patient and humiliation to the surgeon. It is, therefore, imperative that information about high velocity missile wounds and explosive blast injuries should be taught to all medical personnel and, in particular, to surgeons in training.

The Chair of Military Surgery, which I have the honour to hold, was founded in 1860. The first Professor was Sir Thomas Longmore who held the Chair for 31 years and who is regarded as the doyen of teachers in this field; he wrote a book called *Gunshot Wounds* in 1863. This book formed the basis of most teaching for the next 30 years and was widely used in the American Civil War and in the wars of the remaining part of the 19th century. Lt.-Col. Professor W. S. Stevenson was the third

Professor of Military Surgery and his books *Wounds in War, the Mechanism of their Production and their Treatment* was first published in 1897 and the third edition in 1910. He was a pioneer of experimental work in this field on the mechanism of injury in gunshot wounds and the wisdom in its pages is a distillation of the experience of very many surgeons and the enormous number of patients whom they treated.

The Chair of Military Surgery became a Joint Chair with the Royal College of Surgeons in 1960. One of the roles of the Professor is to teach the principles of military surgery to all doctors on entry to the Army and to all the surgeons in training of the Navy, Army and Air Force. During the last five years, the teaching has been extended to the civilian sphere; this has always occurred on a small scale but the time was opportune that it should be taught more widely. I believe that all surgeons in training and those consultants who have no experience of these wounds should be taught the mechanisms of injury and the principles of treatment of high velocity wounds and explosive blast injuries. To that end, we have made enormous strides in the last five years with the very active encouragement of the Presidents of the Royal Colleges of Surgeons, the Association of Surgeons, the Director General of Army Medical Services, the Commandant of the Royal Army Medical College and the Director of Army Surgery. Lectures to the medical schools, postgraduate institutions and postgraduate medical centres have met with an enthusiastic reception and there is obviously an increasing awareness of the problem and increasing demand for instruction on this matter. It is now taught at most Fellowship courses; questions have been asked in the Fellowship written paper and in particular in the *Viva Voce* part of the examination; there are chapters in most of the British surgical textbooks and it would be true to say that the concept of accepting bullet and blast wounds as just another subdivision of trauma about which all medical personnel should know the basic elements has very nearly reached fruition.

The vast respository of knowledge of missile wounds in times of war comes in particular from World War II. Those young surgeons who were drafted into the Medical Services have, by now, retired or will shortly do so. Many of them, over the years, have been particularly involved with the RAMC and have given very freely of their experiences and advice to the Department of Military Surgery and to me in particular. I have drawn very heavily on the experience of the surgeons from that conflict, Palestine, Korea, East Africa, Malaya, Cyprus, Aden, and Northern Ireland. Many of my present and past colleagues have shared their experiences in order that we might improve the scope and quality of the teaching that we give. The enormous experience of the United States in dealing with the wounded from Vietnam has been made freely available, both in the open literature and in discussions with the surgeons concerned. Similarly a close co-operation and interchange of information has been maintained with the surgeons at civilian hospitals in Northern Ireland extending over the last ten years of that conflict.

My hope in writing this book is that it will prove of use to surgeons throughout this country and abroad in teaching the mechanism of injury in high velocity missile wounds and from this understanding will naturally follow the principles of treatment and the details of management of various wounds. My lectures at the Royal Army Medical College, the Royal College of Surgeons and the various postgraduate institutions in this country and abroad have been its basis. I have taken advice from clinicians who have dealt with these wounds in all parts of the world and in many specialist fields I have drawn heavily on their experiences.

No book can cover every eventuality and I recognize that this must be incomplete. If it fulfils the hopes that I have expressed with regard to teaching this subject, then it will have justified its existence; I hope that it will accomplish, in some measure, the task I set myself when I assumed the Chair of Military Surgery. If it reaches a wide audience of those who will be concerned in the future with the management of these wounds, then we in the RAMC will have held faith with those surgeons from the past who were thrown in at the deep end to manage many missile injured patients without adequate instruction as to the principles of treatment and the management required.

War surgery is not a big branch of the surgical tree of knowledge but this may not always be the case; at some time in the future any surgeon may be required to lean heavily on that branch. The principles laid down in this book are based upon the experience of thousands of surgeons on millions of patients. The principles have stood the test of time and must now be accepted into the undergraduate and postgraduate curriculum in perpetuity.

To paraphrase the philosopher Santanya 'Those who do not remember the mistakes of the past are condemned to repeat them'.

M. S. Owen-Smith

London 1981

Acknowledgements

It is a pleasure indeed, to acknowledge the help and advice I have obtained from the surgical veterans of World War II, the honorary consultants to the Army, all my colleagues past and present both within the RAMC and in the civilian field in the UK, the United States of America and Sweden. Most of the research work quoted has been done at the Chemical Defence Establishment at Porton and I am grateful for permission to publish many of the photographs from them. Many of the photographs come from the Slide Library of my Department to which many of my colleagues have contributed and I am grateful for their generosity in permission to publish any of their cases. Figures 1.1 to 1.5 were provided by the National Army Museum and Fig. 2.1b by the Royal Small Arms Factory, Enfield.

My particular thanks go to my secretary, Mrs Christine Squires, for the enormous amount of work in typing and organizing the script and to Tony Allen, Tim Edwards, Phil Ray and Yvonne Miller of the Departments of Photography and Medical Illustration of the Royal Army Medical College for many of the photographs and illustrations.

Finally, I must express my heartfelt thanks to my wife without whose constant help and encouragement this book would never have been written.

M. S. O-S

London, 1981

Contents

Part 3 Regional Management

Part 1
Mechanism of Injury

I
Explosives and guns

Guns

We shall never know for certain who discovered gunpowder. The first man to record the composition was an Englishman, Roger Bacon, a Franciscan friar who studied at Oxford and who wrote *De Secretis Operibus Artis et Naturiae et de Nullitate Magicae* in about 1260. The Chinese certainly had rockets, Roman candles, fire arrows and incendiary grenades in the thirteenth century but there is no evidence that they had gunpowder. There is a similar lack of evidence from India and it is reasonable to believe that two great nations with a wealth of well recorded history would have made note of such a striking phenomenon and there would be material evidence of its existence. Roger Bacon had good reason to be cautious when writing of his scientific knowledge and he recorded the formula for gunpowder in the form of a cypher and anagram hidden in his book. The refinement of crude saltpetre was clearly described and the recipe for gunpowder given as '7 parts of saltpetre, 5 of young hazelwood charcoal and 5 of sulphur'. The method described by him was still being used in Europe in the 1850s, six centuries later.

The invention of the gun came considerably later but again the event is shrouded in some mystery. The popular attribution to Berthold Schwartz in Germany in 1313 is almost certainly mythical and it could be that the use of gunpowder to propel missiles was discovered about the same time by a number of people in the first quarter of the fourteenth century. The first known illustration of a gun appears in an illuminated English manuscript for King Edward III by Walter de Milemete in 1326. The illustration shows a gun, shaped rather like a fat-bodied, narrow-necked vase resting on a wooden bench and with a heavy arrow just being discharged. This gun is remarkably like a bronze cannon found in Loshult, Sweden and since dated about 1300 which is now in the National History Museum in Stockholm. Crude cannon were widely developed in the remaining part of the century and were recorded as being used in battles such as Crecy in 1346. Cannon were made larger and there were inevitable problems with the materials that were used. There were two separate developments in construction, first the casting of larger muzzle-loading cannon from iron and then later in bronze. These developed further and lasted until the nineteenth century in the shape that most people nowadays would recognize. The other method was to use strips of wrought iron around a wooden core or mandrel of circular cross-section, then white-hot iron bands were driven over the tube to strengthen the gun barrel. They had separate breech blocks which could be loaded, fitted into the barrel and held in place by a wedge. Some enormous guns were made in this fashion and examples can still be seen today such as 'Mons Meg' in Edinburgh. Some amazing feats of casting bronze to make huge guns have been recorded. For example the 'Dardanelles Gun' at the Tower of London was cast in 1460 for Muhammed II. It is 17 ft long and weighs nearly 19 tons; it has a calibre of 25 in and fires stone shot weighing 800 lb.

The gun makers also made smaller cannon that could be held in the hands and these 'handguns' developed along separate lines from the heavier pieces. To start with it consisted simply of a metal tube with a hole at the proximal end; this was attached to a wooden staff which was held under the soldier's arm. Gunpowder was poured into the barrel from the muzzle end, followed by a round, lead ball or bullet which fitted into the barrel snugly and which could be rammed into place. When a red hot wire or flame was applied to the touch hole the gunpowder in the barrel ignited and the explosive gases projected a bullet up the barrel as a missile. To overcome the problems of keeping a fire going the slow match was developed, this was a piece of woven cord soaked in a strong solution of saltpetre and then dried. This, when lighted, would continue to burn slowly at about an inch or so a minute. Powder could be placed in a priming pan adjacent to the touch-hole leading through the barrel into the main charge in the gun chamber. This pan sometimes had a cover to stop the powder from blowing away or getting wet. When the gunner was ready to fire he would blow on his slow match before thrusting it into the pan. This method was rather cumbersome and attempts were made to find some means whereby the gun could be fired more easily.

The first piece of mechanical firing device fitted to a gun was the matchlock, 'lock' thereafter being the term used for any form of mechanical firing device. The earliest type was extremely simple; a piece of metal shaped like the letter S was fitted on a pivot to the side of the gun just behind the touch-hole. At the tip of the upper part of the S was a clip into which the glowing end of the slow match could be fitted. The whole moving part was called a serpentine. To fire the weapon, the lower part of the S was pulled backwards and the serpentine arched forward pressing the glowing match tip onto the powder in the priming pan (Fig. 1.1). Such a 'matchlock' weapon was commonly called an arquebus, or other similar corruptions of the French or German language equivalents. By convention the weapons were described in terms of the weight of the projectile; for larger cannon it might be, for example, 8, 16 or 32 lb whereas for the hand-held guns it would be 12, 14 or 16 pure lead balls to the pound and this figure was known as the bore of the gun. The internal diameter of the barrel was called the calibre.

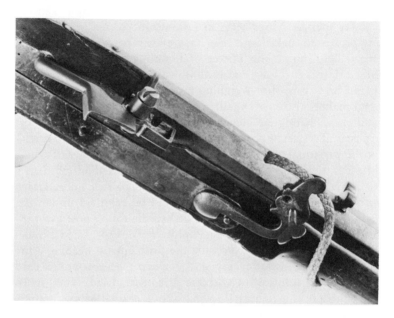

Fig. 1.1 A matchlock musket showing the match and the priming pan which has its cover opened to expose the priming powder.

By the fifteenth century the early hand gun which had consisted of a barrel secured to a simple wooden arm had become far more sophisticated. The wooden body or stock, had acquired something like its modern shape with a butt moulded to fit against the shoulder. By now the weapon was called a matchlock musket and, although it was in widespread use and relatively cheap to produce, it did have its limitations. The musketeer was very much at the mercy of the elements, for rain or wind could extinguish the match or blow away the priming powder. Gun makers made many attempts to produce a weapon which could be loaded and prepared for firing and then put on one side for instant action, requiring no further attention. What they required was a means of ignition and although the idea of producing sparks by striking metal and stone together was an old one and had long been used as a means of making fire, it was not until early in the sixteenth century, probably in Italy, that someone decided to use the same system to ignite the powder in the gun. Pyrites is commonly found in quantity over most of Europe and if struck briskly with a piece of hard metal a plentiful rain of sparks is produced. This was the basis of the new system and so the wheel-lock was developed. This consisted of a steel wheel with its edge grooved and cross-cut connected to a large V-shaped spring.

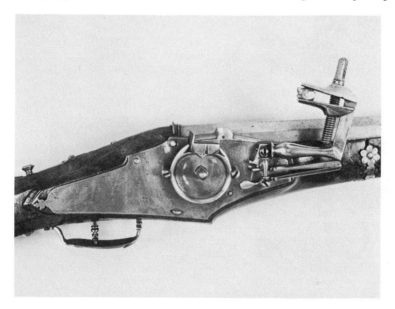

Fig. 1.2 The wheel-lock musket showing the square cut lug by which the spring driving the wheel was wound up. It also shows the arm or dog-head holding a piece of pyrites swung clear of the pan and ready for firing.

The wheel could be turned, thus putting the spring under tension and then locked into place. The wheel was positioned so that its rim formed part of the base of the priming pan. An arm holding a piece of pyrites was now swung forward so that the mineral was pressed into the pan and priming powder; when the trigger was pressed the V-spring was released and rotated the wheel rapidly. The roughened edge of the steel wheel rubbed against the pyrites producing sparks which ignited the priming and fired the main charge. Another advantage of the wheel-lock was that it could be produced in any size and gunsmiths were able to produce weapons small enough to be carried on the person and so the pistol was evolved. However, the system was by no means perfect and prompted the gun makers to search for simpler means of ignition. The wheel-lock's intricate mechanism meant that it was prone to mechanical failure and if a breakage did occur it could only be mended by a gunsmith (Fig. 1.2).

The principle of friction ignition was obviously the correct one but what was needed was a simpler method of obtaining it. Around the middle of the sixteenth century there appeared the first locks using a newer and simpler method known as a Scandinavian or Baltic lock or

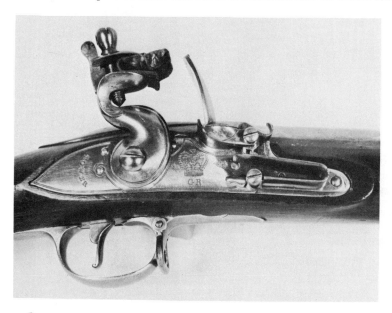

Fig. 1.3 The flintlock musket. The flint is carried on the cock and as it swings forward it will strike sparks from the frizzen at the same time tipping it up on the pivot at the tip of the short arm so exposing the priming and allowing the sparks to fall into the powder.

more commonly the Snaphaunce. This consisted of a spring-loaded mechanism controlling a pivoted arm or cock carrying a flint at its tip. Above the priming pan was a roughened steel plate also on a pivot. If the cock was pulled back and then released by the trigger, the priming pan cover slid open and the arm swung forwards and downwards in an arc, which allowed the flint to scrape down the steel producing sparks. At the same time the pivoted steel was displaced forwards revealing the priming powder which was ignited by the sparks.

The Snaphaunce was closely followed by a further development called the flintlock. The main difference in this mechanism was that the pan cover and the steel were combined into a single L-shaped, pivoted piece of metal known as the frizzen. The action was simple, effective and successful and the basic system remained in common use until the middle of the nineteenth century (Fig. 1.3).

The adoption of the flintlock musket did not affect the system of loading which in most cases was from the muzzle, although a few weapons were loaded through the breech. The problem of estimating the weight of powder to pour into the gun was solved to some extent by the use of prepacked paper cartridges.

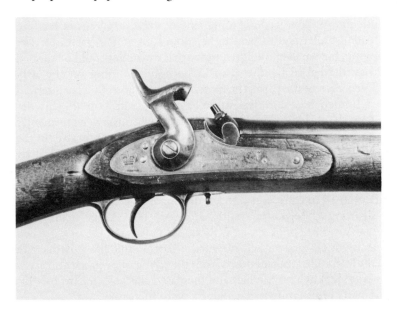

Fig. 1.4 The percussion cap lock for musket or rifle. The percussion cap fits over the small nipple which has a tiny hole through it leading into the breech and so to the charge of powder.

Most of these muskets fired a lead ball weighing 1.3–1.6 oz (35–50 g); muzzle velocities were about 500–1000 ft/s (150–310 m/s) and the musket ball would be projected up to about 400 yards. They were usually used at close quarters in war and most injuries at that time were caused at less than 50 yards range.

Muskets were in use for over three hundred years and were widely used in the wars of Europe culminating at Waterloo, but their action used to be rather uncertain even when the flintlock fired the charge. The flintlock was superceded in 1836 by a lock which could strike a percussion cap made of mercury fulminate which, in turn, fired the gunpowder. The more reliable method was adopted to form the percussion musket. In the English Army the muzzle loading percussion musket was replaced partially by the Minie rifle in 1851 and altogether by the Enfield rifle in 1855 (Fig. 1.4).

Rifles

A system of grooving the musket barrel was invented about 1520, this allowed the lead ball to fit more tightly into the barrel so that the propellent gases from the explosive powder were contained behind the ball and it was projected faster, farther and more accurately. However, the great difficulty in the muzzle-loading rifle was the problems in loading it. The round bullet had to be a tight enough fit in the barrel to take the grooving, but small enough to ensure that the bullet could be pushed right down the barrel by the ramrod without jamming on the way down. Even then with perfectly matched barrel and bullets, repeated firing was limited due to the deposition of fouling from both the powder and lead on the inside of the barrel. These rifled muskets were mainly used as sporting guns but they were used in warfare sporadically. In the American War of Secession the accuracy of the hunting rifles used by the colonists was proven by reports of men being hit at 400 yards. In a trial made in 1924 using some of these eighteenth century muzzle-loading rifles of 0.4–0.45 in calibre at 300 yards range, five hits out of ten on a man-size target were consistently attained. The simple device discovered in America about 1725 (Wilson, 1921) was the use of a greased cloth patch which was pushed down the barrel after the powder and cleared the lead and carbon deposits from the rifling. The patch also acted as a gas-tight seal behind the ball and increased the velocity up to 1800 ft/s (550 m/s). Thus range and accuracy were increased.

The major advance in design was in 1841 when Delvigne showed that elongated lead bullets with a hollow in the base had their bases expanded into the grooves of the barrel by the pressure of the powder gas. Bullets of this shape could easily pass down the barrel whilst the expansion of their base, ensured their taking the grooving. In 1847 Captain Minie modified the hollow bullet by inserting an iron cup in the base, as this made the expansion of the base more certain and symmetrical. The new bullets were used in the existing, rifled, muzzle-loading percussion musket and the combination called the Minie rifle. Some of the English Army in the Crimea in 1854 were armed with these weapons and they were proven to be so superior to the smooth bore musket that the whole army was supplied with the newer and even more effective fire-arm in 1855. This was the Enfield three-grooved rifle which fired an expanding cylindroconoidal bullet of 0.55 in calibre, weighing 34 g, at a velocity of 1200 ft/s (370 m/s) (Fig 1.5).

Many minor improvements were made but the next major invention

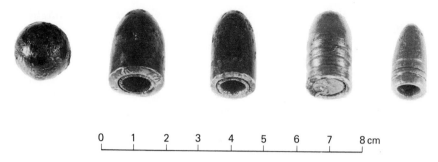

Fig. 1.5 British Service Ammunition – bullets. Reading from left to right they are: 1. Spherical musket ball; 2. Minie bullet (cylindroconoidal, hollow base, iron cup); 3. Enfield bullet (cyclindroconoidal, hollow base, iron cup, later replaced by box wood and clay plugs); 4. Snider-Enfield boxer bullet (cylindroconoidal, hollow base, clay plug, three cannelures hollow tip); 5. Mk 2 Webley bullet (cylindroconoidal, hollow base, three cannelures). This last bullet was in use up until the beginning of World War II. The more recent design of military bullets are shown in Fig. 2.1.

was that of breech loading using metal cartridges and most countries adopted this principle for their army rifles. New rifles incorporating these changes were made; new propellants such as blackpowder and cordite raised the muzzle velocities up to 2000 ft/s (615 m/s); the calibre was reduced to less than 0.315 in (8 mm) and to withstand the stresses, the bullets were coated with a hard gilding metal like cupronickel. Magazines carrying up to ten cartridges enabled rapid fire to take place and so by the turn of the century the rifles were much as we know them today and had a similar wounding capacity. The 1898 Mauser 8.22 mm for example, had a muzzle velocity of 2900 ft/s (878 m/s) which is in excess of the standard NATO 7.62 mm rifle used today.

The high velocity bullet is, therefore, not new but the effects of it have been such that in each war since about 1850 accusations have been made that explosive bullets have been used. As the velocity of bullets increased in the latter half of the nineteenth century, surgeons with an active interest in bullet wounds investigated the mechanism of injury. It was readily proven that bullets do not have to be filled with explosives for the effect on tissues to be apparently similar to that of an explosion.

High velocity bullet wounds

The wounds from musket balls have been well described by Paré, Wiseman, John Hunter, Larrey, Guthrie, Hennen and Sir Charles Bell. Ambroise Paré wrote 'Verily neither a stag with his horns, nor a flint out of a sling can give so great a blow or make so large a wound as a leaden or iron bullet shot out of a gun, as that which going with mighty violence pierces the body like a thunderbolt'. Stevenson in 1897 wrote 'The old round bullet at its highest rate of velocity, made an entrance wound in the skin the edges of which were surrounded by a wide area of contusion. The skin wound produced by this missile showed a distinct evidence of loss of substance, a circular portion of about the same diameter as the bullet itself being punched out, the edges of the aperture being inverted. The track through the soft parts was much lacerated and contused and its diameter was usually greater than that of the bullet. The exit wound was always greater in extent than on the entrance side, it hardly ever showed the punched out appearance seen in the entrance wound, but was formed of triangular flaps of skin everted, evidently burst outward by a pressure from within.'

There is little doubt that many of these wounds were severe with a high mortality and morbidity and most were received at relatively close range. All the energy of the ball was utilized in creating a wound as its large size and surface area caused great retardation. If a long bone was broken it was usually only into a few pieces and commonly the ball was squashed against the bone. If it struck flat bone the ball would usually perforate leaving a fairly regular hole with some comminution surrounding it.

The wounds of high velocity bullets from the rifled muskets were first noticed by Huguier (1848) who postulated the hydrodynamic theory of wounding to explain how the tissues were displaced and damaged widely at a distance from the bullet itself. These more severe wounds were commented on by a number of observers, in particular in the massive, classical record in three volumes of the *Medical and Surgical History of the American Civil War* by Otis (1870, 1876), and by Longmore (1877). Surgeons in England, Germany and France began detailed studies of the physical effects of the bullets on inanimate material, on animals and human cadavers to find an explanation of the wounds seen on the battlefield.

The earliest experiments in this important field were developed in the 1870s and Kocher published the first significant report of experimental observation on wounds from high velocity projectiles in 1875. By the turn of the century most of the effects of bullets travelling at velocities of up to 2400 ft/s (740 m/s) were known. Observers like Bruns, von Coler, Demosthen, Delorme, Chavasse, Stevenson, Keith and Rigby demonstrated wounds in the carcasses of animals and in human cadavers both at simulated and real ranges. They correlated these wounds with human wounds caused in battle. In 1894 Sir Victor Horsley gave a masterly lecture at the Royal Institution which was entitled *The Destructive Effects of Small Projectiles*. He disposed of a number of theories as to how bullets caused a wound and he ascribed wounding power to the transmission of energy from the bullet to the particles of the tissues which are hurried forward' and in effect increased the size of the projectile. He discussed the effects of the penetrating bullet on tissues of different consistency referring to the work of Huguier in 1848 who suggested that the 'lateral disturbance' in soft tissue was a hydrodynamic effect. Horsley's experience in anaesthetized dogs confirmed such an effect on the brain as the cause of cessation of respiration when a bullet passed through the head. He demonstrated the physical consequences of the passage of a bullet by firing into soap and clay and measuring the variation in the diameter of the projectile track as related to its velocity. Lt-Col. Professor Stevenson was a successor to Sir Thomas Longmore as Professor of Military Surgery at Netley. In 1897 he published his book in which he described experiments in which he fired bullets through open and closed lead cans filled with water and demonstrated that the hydrodynamic effect was not due to the shock wave but began after the bullet had passed through the can. The visible effects were often greater on the entry rather than the exit side of the cans, and he referred to similar results by von Coler in Germany. (Photographs of the disrupted cans were shown in his book and the specimens kept in the Royal Army Medical College Museum until destroyed in the London blitz) (Figs. 1.6, 1.7, 1.8).

In 1898 Woodruff referred to these European experiments and suggested the word 'cavitation' to describe the physical phenomenon whereby energy is transferred from the bullet to the tissues to cause damage at a distance from the bullet track.

The turn of the century saw a flurry of reports on bullet wound experiments and conflicting results were sometimes obtained. The Prussian War Ministry organized a massive programme of research using cadavers in which bullets were fired at full charge at ranges from 25 to 2000 yards. One thousand preparations were preserved in the Friedrick Wilhelm Institute in Berlin and the more important ones reproduced as full size illustrations in an atlas issued by the Ministry (MacCormac, 1895).

The South African war, the Spanish-American war and World War I produced many unjustified charges of the use of explosive bullets. The experienced war surgeon had seen it all before and did not draw any distinction between the wounds caused by any of the rifles of the day. Professor Stevenson summed up the position of most military surgeons when he wrote 'So much has been written, since small bore rifles have been invented on the so-called explosive effects of rifle bullets, that one might almost be led to believe that this class of wound is an outcome of the use of the modern bullet of small calibre, and that these extensive

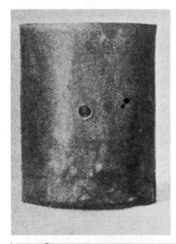

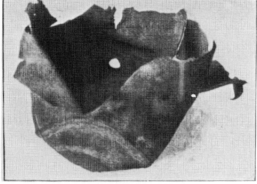

Fig. 1.6 Empty lead vessel showing aperture of bullet (RAM College Museum).

Fig. 1.7 Lead vessel filled with water and sealed showing effect of the rifle bullet (RAM College Museum).

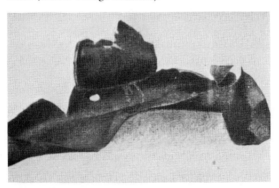

Fig. 1.8 Lead vessel filled with water and left open showing effect of rifle bullet (RAM College Museum).

injuries were a new feature in gun-shot wounds, whereas quite the contrary is the fact. The severity of the explosive effect is, if anything, greater with the older rifle bullets than it is with the new'.

Little genuine progress in the field of wound ballistics was made after World War I until the extensive work of Callender and French in 1935. World War II produced an immediate expansion of interest in research and for the first time the cavitation process was demonstrated photographically by Black, Burns and Zuckerman in 1941. Since that time extensive research work in the USA, England, Sweden, Germany and Yugoslavia has clarified many of the problems of wound ballistics. The subject has now grown into a science in its own right, with international meetings and exchange of research findings. There are still some problems left unsolved but much research continues to elucidate these and to push back the frontiers of knowledge to promote further understanding of the mechanisms by which missiles cause wounds, and thereby improve the treatment of patients wounded by these agents.

References and Further Reading

Bernal Diaz (1963). *The Conquest of New Spain.* (Trans. J. M. Cohen), Penguin Classics, London.

Black, A. N., Burns, B. D. and Zuckerman, S. (1941). An experimental study of the wounding mechanism of high velocity missiles. *British Medical Journal*, **2**, 872–874.

Blackmore, H.L. (1961). *British Military Firearms 1650–1850.* Herbert Jenkins, London.

Blackmore, H.L. (1971). *Hunting Weapons.* Barrie and Jenkins, London.

Callender, G.R. and French, R.W. (1935). Wound ballistics – studies in the mechanism of wound production by rifle bullets. *The Military Surgeon*, **77**, 177–201.

Editorial (1899). Professor von Brun's experiments. *Lancet*, **1**, 319.

Greener, W.W. (1910). *The Gun and its Development.* Facsimile 10th Edn, Arms and Armour Press, Lionel Leventhal Ltd, London.

Guthrie, G.J. (1815). *On Gunshot Wounds of the Extremities.* Longman, London.

Hennen, J. (1818). *Observations on some Important Points in the Practice of Military Surgery.* Constable, Edinburgh.

Horsley, V. (1894). The destructive effects of small projectiles. Nature **50**, 104–108.

Huguier, M. (1848). Plaies d'armes à feu. *Bulletin de l'Academie Nationale de Medicine*, **14**, 7–112.

Hunter, J. (1794). *A Treatise on the Blood, Inflammation and Gunshot Wounds.* G. Nicholl, London.

Keith, A. and Rigby, H.H. (1899). Modern military bullets, a study of their destructive effects. *Lancet*, **2**, 1499–1507.

Kocher, T. (1875) Uber die Sprengwirkung der modernen Kleingewehr-Gesthosse. *Correspondenz-Blatt für Schweizer Aerzte*, **3**, 29–33.

Longmore, T. (1877). *Gunshot Injuries*. Longmans Green & Co., London.

MacCormac, N. (1895). Some points of interest in connection with the surgery of war. *Lancet*, **2**, 290–2.

Otis, G.A. (1870, 1876). *The Medical and Surgical History of the War of Rebellion*. Government Printing Office, Washington.

Singer, D.W. (1924). *Selected Works of Ambroise Paré*. Medical Classics Series. John Bale, Sons and Danillson Ltd., London.

Stevenson, W.F. (1897). *Wounds in War: The Mechanism of their Production and Treatment*. Longmans Green & Co. London.

Textbook of Small Arms (1929). HMSO, London.

Wilson, L.B. (1921). Dispersion of bullet energy in relation to wound effects. *The Military Surgeon*, **49**, 241–51.

Wiseman, R. (1705). *Eight Chirurgical Treatises*, 4th Edn, B. Tooke and J. Meredith, London.

Woodruff, C.E. (1898). The causes of the explosive effects of modern small calibre bullets. *New York Medical Journal*, **67**, 593–601.

2

Wound ballistics

Wound ballistics is defined as the study of the motion of missiles within the body and the wounding capacity of various missiles (Fig. 2.1a, 2.1b).

The study of bullet wounds requires knowledge of the behaviour of the bullet after it has been discharged from the breech of a gun and the effect it has on the tissues it penetrates. The motion of the bullet in flight and within the tissues after impact depend on several variable factors. These include the size, shape, composition, and above all, the velocity and stability of the bullet. In the tissues the elasticity and the density are the most important factors which influence the retardation of the penetrating missile.

During World War II, Black, Burns and Zuckerman (1941) were able to demonstrate the effects of high velocity missiles on gelatine blocks and rabbit legs using spark shadow-photography. Since then high speed cinematography and high intensity x-ray exposures at millionths of a second duration have been used to provide detailed information of these effects.

The shape of a missile is important; the more irregular the shape of the missile the more liable it will be to tumble in the air with consequent loss of range and accuracy. Some missiles like arrows and darts are inherently stable. This is because the centre of the resistance to flight is placed in the feathers and this lies well behind the centre of gravity of the missile as a whole. An arrow, if fired into the air, will eventually come down point first. Other missiles like bullets are basically unstable. The long bullet of the rifle is designed to be the optimum shape for a missile travelling above the speed of sound; the centre of resistance to flight lies at the nose of the bullet whereas the centre of gravity lies well behind it. Such a missile is inherently unstable, and thus the bullet in flight tends to oscillate around its long axis. This important deviation is known as yaw and in the extremes of this motion the bullet may, indeed, tumble end over end. Spinning the bullet by means of the rifling in the barrel gives it stability and this increases its range and accuracy; this spin induces other variations in motion of the bullet so that it performs a fairly complicated pattern of deviation from the line of its long

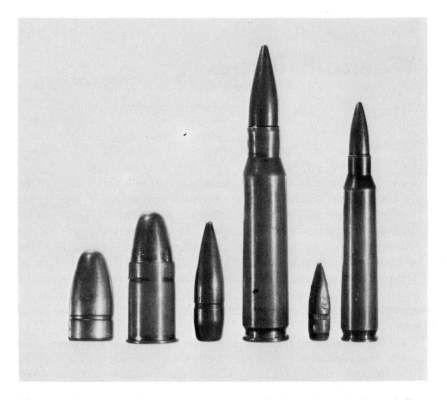

Fig. 2.1a A comparison between the appearance of a low velocity hand gun bullet and high velocity rifle bullets. On the left is the 0.45 in bullet, alone and also in its small cartridge case. In the centre is the 7.62 mm and on the right the 5.56 mm rifle bullet, each of them alone and also in its cartridge case. The high velocity rifle bullets show the relatively small sized bullet and the very long cartridge case, containing a large amount of propellant, when compared with the low velocity bullet.

axis (Fig. 2.2). Precession is a circular yaw about the centre of gravity which takes the shape of a decreasing spiral. Nutation is a rotational movement in small circles which forms a rosette pattern like a spinning top. Irregular movements are rapidly damped by the gyroscopic action of the spin at up to 3500 revolutions per second and this action tends to stabilize the bullet in flight after about 100 metres. After this the bullet will fly true and we must remember that these rifle bullets are used for accurate target shooting at ranges of 1000 metres, and sometimes more, and have been known to kill at a range of up to 2 miles. However, the spin is inadequate to maintain stability of the bullet in media that are denser than air. Now the soft tissues of the body and of water are 800–

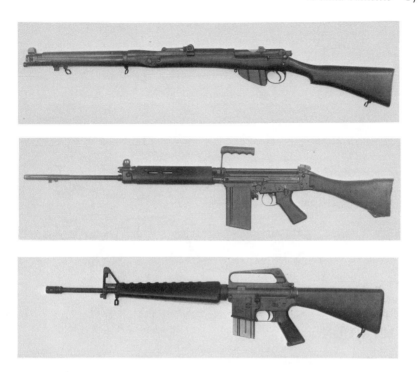

Fig. 2.1b Some typical rifles: *Top:* Lee-Enfield 0.303 in bullet weighs 11.7 g muzzle velocity 780 m/s (2540 ft/s); *Centre:* FN SLR 7.62 mm bullet weighs 9.4 g; muzzle velocity 860 m/s (2790 ft/s); *Bottom:* Colt Armalite M 16 5.56 mm bullet weighs 3.6 g; muzzle velocity 980 m/s (3185 ft/s).

900 times as dense as air and when a bullet hits these tissues it always becomes unstable; any angle of yaw that is present will be greatly increased, with deviation from its straight course and an increase in tissue retardation and consequent damage.

A wound results from the absorbtion of energy imparted by a missile when it strikes and penetrates tissue. Its available kinetic energy is calculated by the formula $KE = MV^2/2$ where M represents the mass and V the velocity. This means that doubling the mass would double the energy available, whereas doubling the velocity will quadruple the energy (Fig. 2.3). When M is in kg and V is m/s, then KE is measured in joules.

When a missile is stopped by the tissues it penetrates, then the energy liberated to cause damage must be equal to the total KE of the missile. If it passes through the tissues it has a remaining velocity from which can be calculated the energy released during wounding.

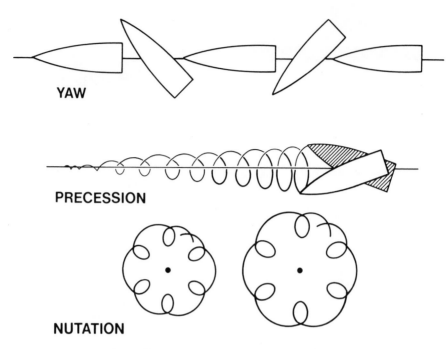

Fig. 2.2 Yaw is the oscillation around the long axis of the bullet. Precession is a circular yaw about the centre of gravity which takes the shape of a decreasing spiral. Nutation is a rotational movement in a small circle which forms a rosette pattern like a spinning top.

$$\text{Energy expended} = \frac{M(V_1{}^2 - V_2{}^2)}{2}$$

where V_1 = strike velocity and V_2 = remaining velocity.

The lower this remaining velocity, the greater the proportion of the kinetic energy that has been liberated to the tissues. The retardation of the missile is an important factor in the creation of the wound and it depends upon a number of missile factors, already described and also on a number of tissue factors of which the most important are the tissue density and the elasticity. Kocher in 1876 demonstrated that tissues which contain large quantities of water are most severely damaged, and Daniel in 1944 correlated high velocity missile damage with the specific gravity of the tissue involved.

Mechanism of injury

A bullet can cause injury in the following three ways depending upon its velocity.

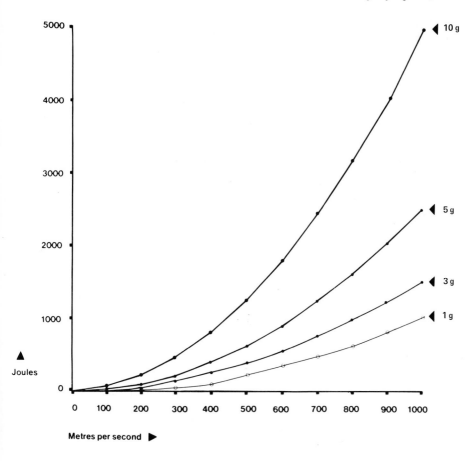

Kinetic energy at different velocities

Fig. 2.3 The effect of increasing velocity on the kinetic energy of missiles of different masses.

Laceration and crushing

As the missile penetrates the tissues they are crushed and forced apart. This is the principal effect of low velocity missiles travelling at up to 1100 ft/s (340 m/s). The crushing and laceration caused solely by the passage of the missile is not serious unless vital organs or major blood vessels are injured directly by the missile. Only those tissues that have come into immediate contact with the missile are damaged and the wound is comparable to those caused by hand held weapons such as knives. No significant energy is transmitted to the tissues surrounding the wound track; the damage seen at operation is all the damage and nothing is

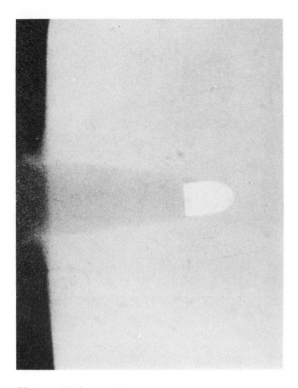

Fig. 2.4 High speed photograph of a low velocity 0.45 in bullet entering a block of 20 per cent gelatin. Low velocity bullets simply core out a track in the tissue with minimal displacement. This is shown in diagramatic form in Fig. 2.5 with a 0.38 in low velocity bullet fired through a block of 20 per cent gelatin.

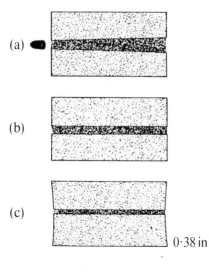

(a)

(b)

(c)

0·38 in

Fig. 2.5 Drawings of selected frames from a 16 mm cine film taken with a high speed camera at 8000 frames per second. The block is made of 20 per cent gelatin. a. A 0.38 in bullet at 200 m/s (660 ft/s), penetrating the block and coring out a track by displacement of the gelatin; b. the track after the bullet has left the block; c. the narrow permanent track which this low velocity bullet has created.

hidden. Figure 2.4 shows a high-speed photograph of a low velocity bullet entering a block of 20 per cent gelatine. The bullet simply cores out a track with minimal displacement of the gelatine and it is rapidly stopped within the block as its small amount of energy is used up in displacing the gelatine against the elastic resistance of the medium (Fig. 2.5).

The other two phenomena occur so quickly that they can only be demonstrated using very high-speed photography or radiography. They only occur at velocities exceeding the speed of sound in air which is approximately 1100 ft/s (340 m/s) and this figure conveniently divides bullets into low or high velocity.

Shock waves

Whilst forcing a track through solid tissues the missile compresses the medium in front of it and this region of compression moves away as a shock wave of spherical form (Figs 2.6, 2.7). This was first demonstrated by Mach and by Boys in 1893 using spark shadow photography. The velocity of the shock wave is approximately that of the velocity of sound in water (4800 ft/s or 1500 m/s) and although the changes of pressure due to shock waves only last about a millionth of a second they may reach peak values of up to 100 atm or 1500 lbf/in^2 (10^6kg/m^2; 10350 kPa)*. Thus they can cause damage at a considerable distance from the permanent wound track. Solid tissues like muscle, liver, spleen and brain are very susceptible and they are conducted particularly well along fluid filled tubes like arteries and veins to cause damage at a distance.

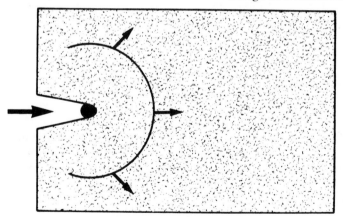

Fig. 2.6 Diagram of a high velocity sphere penetrating a gelatin block. Ahead of the bullet a shock wave of spherical form is transmitted at a velocity of about 1500 m/s (4800 ft/s).

*1 atm≈ 101 kPa; 1 lbf/in ^{2} ≈ 6.9 kPa

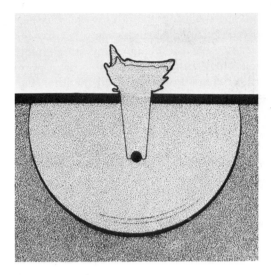

Fig. 2.7 Drawing of a high speed photograph of a spherical bullet travelling at 460 m/s (1500 ft/s) penetrating water. A splash occurs on the surface and the missile creates a conical cavity as it is retarded by the water. Ahead of the bullet travels a shock wave of spherical form.

Temporary cavitation

This phenomenon is encountered only with high velocity missiles and is the main factor in their immensely destructive effects. As the penetrating missile releases its energy rapidly, it is absorbed by the local tissues which are accelerated violently forwards and outwards. Due to their imparted velocity and their momentum the tissues continue to move after the passage of the missile and thus a large cavity is created approximately 30–40 times the diameter of the missile (Figs 2.8 and 2.9). This cavity has a subatmospheric pressure and is connected to the outside by entry and exit holes; therefore, bacteria from the outside, together with clothing and debris, are actively sucked into the depth of the wound. The cavity reaches the maximum size in a few milliseconds and then collapses in a pulsatile fashion leaving a narrow permanent cavity, which is the cavity that may be seen at operation. The high velocity missile shears cleanly through the tissues involved; it is the cavitation effect which results from the rapid transfer of energy from the missile to the tissues which is the mechanism whereby severe wounds are caused. Cavitation takes place mainly after the passage of the missile, and accounts for the 'explosive' nature of high velocity missile wounds. The greater the energy that is imparted to the tissues, the greater is the size of the temporary cavity and the more extensive the damage. Soft tissue will be pulped, small blood vessels will be disrupted and bone may be

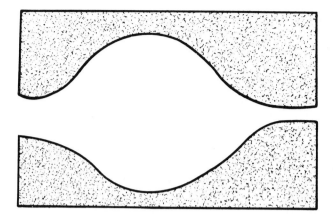

Fig. 2.8 Diagram of the maximum size of the temporary cavity in gelatin block immediately after a high velocity bullet has passed through it.

shattered without being hit directly. The larger blood vessels and nerves being more elastic may be pushed aside, but the blood vessels may well suffer damage of the intima at a distance from the wound even though there are no external signs of injury. Thrombosis and stasis in vessels in the hours following the cavitation injury further increases the volume of dead tissue, plasma leaks from the damaged vessels causing a tense

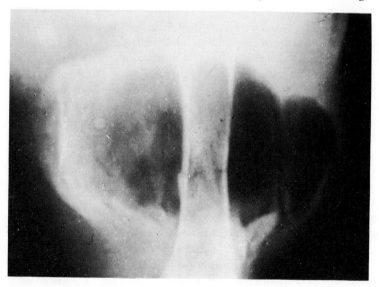

Fig. 2.9 Microsecond radiograph of a thigh of an anaesthetized sheep, showing a temporary cavity caused by a missile travelling at 770 m/s (2500 ft/s). (Crown Copyright Reserved).

oedema and further compressive ischaemia. This large amount of dead tissue, innoculated with bacteria and debris actively sucked in from the environment, is the specific pathological entity of the high velocity missile injury.

The cavitation phenomenon takes place in all tissues whether they be the limb, the abdomen, chest or head. Some tissues such as muscle, liver, brain and the more solid homogeneous organs in general, are very susceptible to damage by this mechanism, whereas others such as lung tissue, which is of lesser density than these, is far more resistant to such damage.

The temporary cavity lasts only a few milliseconds and can only be recorded by very high speed cameras or x-ray exposures of very short duration (1–2 ms) and high intensity (2–300 kV, 2000 A). Twenty per cent gelatine gel simulates soft tissue in its physical properties and is used as a transparent medium. Experimentally a spherical steel bullet may be used as the missile, as this removes the complicating properties of spin, yaw and tumble. A series of stills from such a high-speed cine film at 8000 frames per second is shown in Figs 2.10 and 2.11. The missile is a steel sphere 5 mm (3/16 in) diameter weighing 2 g with a velocity of 1500 ft/s (460 m/s). The stills read from top left downwards and then in sequence and the time is shown in milliseconds. On penetrating the block the cavity is conical in shape with a tail splash of gelatine ejected backwards. Penetrating further, the diameter of the cavity diminishes as the missile's velocity decreases and the shape of the cavity becomes more fusiform. The ball then emerges and leaves the geletine block in just under 2 ms pushing some gelatine ahead of it as a head cone. All the cavitation changes on the rest of the film take place after the bullet has left the block. The temporary cavity then collapses rapidly in pulsatile fashion ending with violent displacement of the whole block.

When the velocity is increased to 2500 ft/s (770 m/s) the cavitation changes are much more marked. In Fig. 2.12 the stills from the high-speed film read from top left across the figure and then in sequence. You will see that the ball has penetrated and left the gelatine block in under 0.5 ms. All the gross cavitation changes that are shown in the rest of the slide take place after the bullet has left the block. In this case the much greater energy transfer from the missile to the gelatine block has caused an enormous cavity and the elasticity of the gelatine has not been able to absorb this transfer. Gelatine is blasted out from the exit face, the whole block is distorted and even at 30 ms the cavitation is still occurring whilst the whole block is lifted up from its base.

Naked eye inspection of such a block afterwards (Fig. 2.13) shows only the narrow permanent track with a few fissures radiating from it. This gives no indication of the violent distortion which has occurred and which is shown in these stills from a cine film. With very high velocity

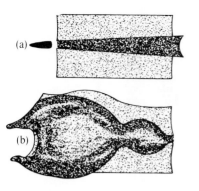

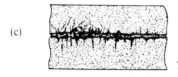

(a)

(b)

(c)

7·62 mm

Fig. 2.10 Drawing of selected frames from high speed cine film of a 7.62 mm rifle bullet passing through a gelatin block at 800 m/s (2600 ft/s). **a.** The bullet just leaving the block and the temporary cavity developing; **b.** the maximum size of the temporary cavity which has grossly distorted the whole block and the ejection of gelatin from the exit face; **c.** the narrow permanent track with a few fissures.

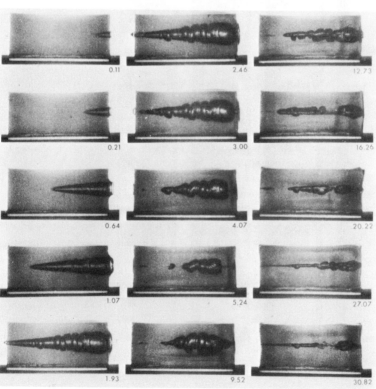

Fig. 2.11 Selected stills from a high speed cine film showing the temporary cavitation from a steel sphere 3/16 in in diameter and weighing 2 g at a velocity of 460 m/s (1500 ft/s). The simulant is a standard gelatin block. (Crown Copyright Reserved)

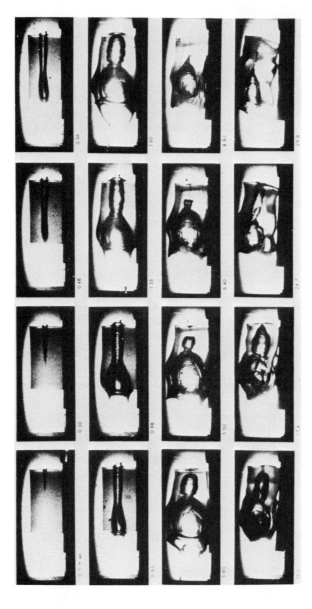

Fig. 2.12 A series of stills from a high speed film of the temporary cavitation from a steel sphere 3/16 in diameter and weighing 2 g at a velocity of 770 m/s (2500 ft/s). The simulant is a standard gelatin block. (Crown Copyright Reserved)

missiles travelling at above 2500 ft/s (770 ms) the elasticity of the surrounding tissues may not be able to contain the cavitation and the effect truly becomes explosive.

Another medium that closely resembles human tissue is soap and this is used experimentally to make permanent records of the size of the temporary cavity. Soap is a plastic medium and, in this case, the maximum size of the temporary cavity is permanently left in the block as an irregularly shaped cavity. This block can then be cut longitudinally thus creating a permanent and easily demonstrable record of the effect of the missile (Fig. 2.14). High-speed and serial radiographs can be made of missile passings through either gelatine or soap blocks at any stage in the development of the cavity. From these studies we know that the greater

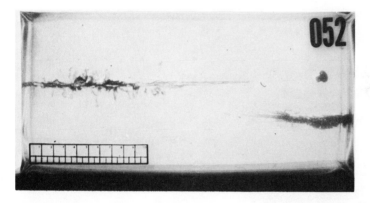

Fig. 2.13 Appearance of the gelatin block afterwards, to show the narrow permanent track with a few fissures radiating from it. (Crown Copyright Reserved)

the retardation of the missile, usually because of increasing angle of yaw or of break up of the missile causing a greater projected surface area, the greater will be the maximum diameter of the cavity which is directly proportional to the energy released.

High-speed cine film or high-speed cine x-ray can demonstrate cavitation in the tissues of the anaesthetized experimental animal and there is a close correlation between cavitation in animal tissue and in the simulants that are used experimentally.

Additional evidence that there has been a temporary cavity is demonstrated by the zone of bruising which occurs around the permanent track of the experimental wound. This is due to the stretching and consequent rupture of small blood vessels by the pressure from the rapidly expanding temporary cavity. This zone of damaged muscle has an abnormal colour, does not contract when pinched and does not bleed when cut.

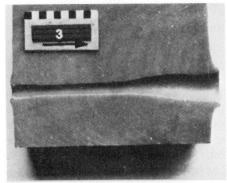

a. The cavitation of a 9 mm bullet fired from a pistol at point blank range.

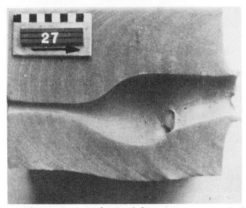

b. The cavitation obtained from a 5.56 mm rifle bullet at 100 m.

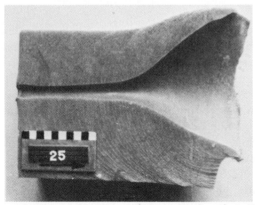

c. The cavitation obtained from a 7.62 mm rifle bullet at 100 m.

Fig. 2.14 The permanent record of cavitation effects as shown in standard soap blocks.

These appearances are characteristic, can be readily demonstrated to the uninitiated and are a fairly accurate estimate of the death of muscle (Fig. 2.15).

Some tissues are much more sensitive to the cavitational changes than others. In general, the damage is directly proportional to the density of the tissue: homogeneous tissues like muscle, liver, spleen and brain are very sensitive, whereas the light tissues such as the lung, which is mainly filled with air, are resistant. The damage is also inversely proportional to the amount of elastic fibres present in the tissue – for example, skin and lung are remarkably resistant to such damage, whereas bone is very sensitive.

Pistol bullets have a relatively low amount of energy available to cause damage; in general this occurs only at fairly close ranges and the damaging effects are very limited at ranges of more than 50–100 metres. All rifle bullets have an incredible amount of available energy, and although this energy decreases with increasing range, nevertheless they have great wounding power, even at distances of many hundreds of metres. If a rifle bullet is stable on impact, it might go right through the limb giving up only 10–20 per cent of its energy. If, however, it becomes unstable it may give up 60–70 per cent of its energy with a consequently much more severe wound.

If the bullet fragments on impact, all the energy will be used up in creating horrendous wounds. The external appearance of a bullet wound can be deceptive. If the bullet enters or leaves skin end-on, then it will commonly leave a small hole, irrespective of the severe damage it may have caused during its passage through the tissues; if the bullet enters or, more commonly, leaves the skin sideways-on to some degree, then the hole in the skin will be large and ragged.

For the same amount of total energy expended, the design of the bullet can make profound differences in its effect on tissues. If the bullet is soft, it will flatten on impact, producing a much greater surface area and, therefore, greater retardation. This design will produce a very early release of energy (Fig. 2.16a). If it is an unstable jacketed bullet, the energy would be more rapidly released as the bullet starts to yaw and tumble (Fig. 2.16b).

If it is a stable jacketed bullet, the energy would tend to be released rather late as the bullet traverses a greater length of tissue and it only becomes unstable with the longer wound track (Fig. 2.16c). The length of the 'neck' or narrow part of the wound track is a measure of the stability of the bullet in soft tissue.

In an experimental rifle bullet wound, a volume of tissue approximately 500 ml (1pt) the size of a fist, is damaged. This large amount of dead tissue, uniformly and grossly contaminated with bacteria and debris

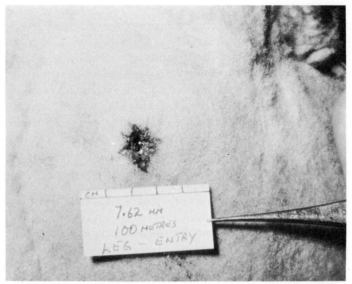

a. Entry wound, 7.62 mm rifle bullet at 100 m on the anaesthetized sheep's thigh.

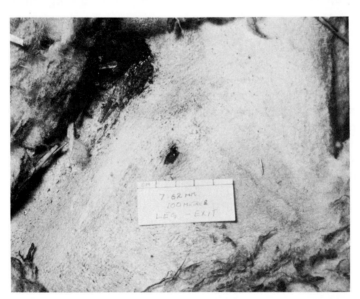

b. Small exit wound.

Fig. 2.15 a–c These photographs show how relatively small entry and exit wounds from a high velocity bullet may conceal enormous damage. (Crown Copyright Reserved).

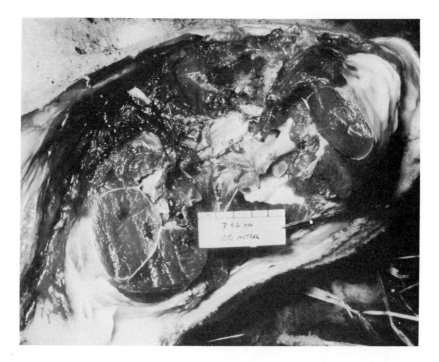

Fig. 2.15 c. Cavitational damage to the thigh at operation. There is a grossly cominuted fracture of the femur with fragments of bone scattered round the periphery of the temporary cavity and a large amount of dead muscle present at the top of the picture.

from the surface, is the pathological entity of the high velocity missile wound.

The larger arteries and veins are violently forced aside during the formation of the cavity but because of their elasticity they are less liable to major damage. However, thrombosis can be caused in a vessel which is apparently intact, and vessels which have been divided may have microscopic evidence of damage for up to 1 cm from the divided end (Fig. 2.17).

The cavitational phenomenon takes place whenever a high velocity bullet enters the abdomen, thorax or head, as well as the limbs.

When the high velocity bullet penetrates the abdomen, not only is a large temporary cavity formed with gross displacement and damage of the viscera, but there is also an effect on gas contained within certain viscera. The pressure wave causes the contained gas to be compressed and then violently expanded, so that the walls of the viscus may be ruptured from within, even if the bullet does not actually penetrate it.

There is an extraordinary difference in the wounding effects of bullets

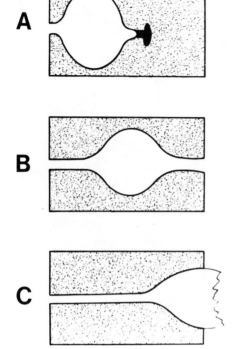

Fig. 2.16 Diagrams of gelatin blocks showing how the design and instability of the bullet influences the size and position of the temporary cavity. **a.** Soft lead bullet, which flattens on impact and gives early release of energy; **b.** relatively unstable, jacketed, military rifle bullet, giving up its energy after penetrating about 5 cm; **c.** stable, jacketed rifle bullet, tending to remain stable until about 10 cm penetration.

striking the abdominal contents at different velocities. The damage to an anaesthetized pig's colon by a bullet fired at 800 ft/s (250 m/s) is two small holes 3 mm by 5 mm with no surrounding haemorrhage (Fig. 2.18). This is the sort of damage which occurs at point-blank range from a pistol bullet. The damage is straight-forward, is equivalent to a simple perforation of the colon and may be treated by conventional surgical methods with success. The same type of bullet fired at 500 m/s (1600 ft/s) causes much larger holes nearly 2 cm in diameter and these holes are surrounded by a zone of obvious bruising (Fig. 2.19).

Microscopically, this zone of damaged tissue extends 2 cm from the edges of the frank perforations. This tissue is dead, and attempts to suture through it will result in disaster. The damaged tissues must be widely excised back to tissues which are healthy, and it may be necessary to resect a portion of colon in order to be well clear of the cavitational injury.

At 770 m/s (2500 ft/s), which is equivalent to an injury from a rifle bullet at about 100 m, the effect is disastrous. In this case, the colon is disrupted and there are microscopic changes of cell death extending 20 cm from the edge of the hole in the colon; this is why such an area

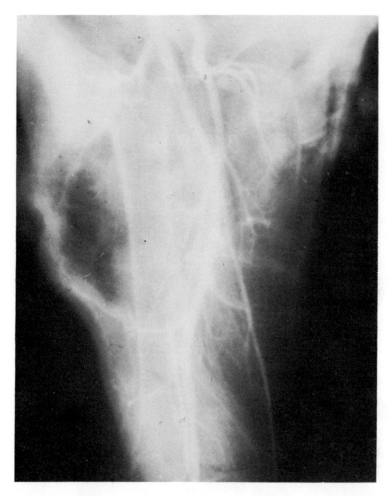

Fig. 2.17 Arteriogram of the anaesthetized sheep's thigh taken at the moment of wounding showing the temporary cavity and the gross displacement of the femoral artery. (Crown Copyright Reserved)

must be resected if it has been damaged by a rifle bullet. No attempts at local repair will be successful in this type of injury from a high–velocity bullet wound of the colon (Fig. 2.20).

The thorax behaves differently from the abdomen, for it is largely filled with air due to the large volume of the chest which is occupied by the lungs. Therefore, as the tissues are not mainly liquid-like, the conditions for the formation of the temporary cavity are not met. The heart and great vessels, being filled with fluid, are extremely susceptible to damage from cavitation and such injuries from a rifle bullet are fatal.

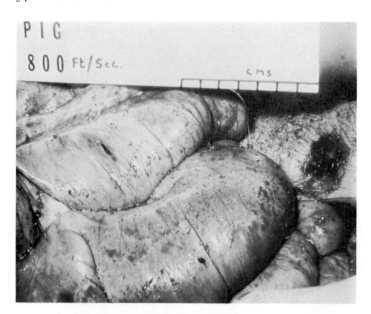

Fig. 2.18 Holes 5 mm in diameter in the anaesthetized pig's colon caused by a standard bullet fired at 250 m/s (800 ft/s). (Crown Copyright Reserved)

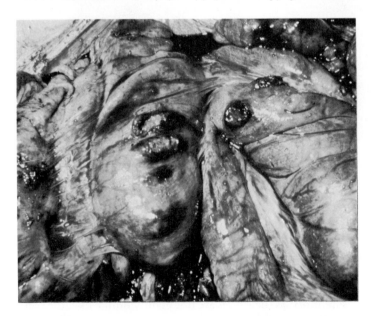

Fig. 2.19 Holes 2 cm in diameter and surrounded by an area of obvious bruising in the anaesthetized pig's colon caused by a standard bullet fired at 500 m/s (1600 ft/s). (Crown Copyright Reserved)

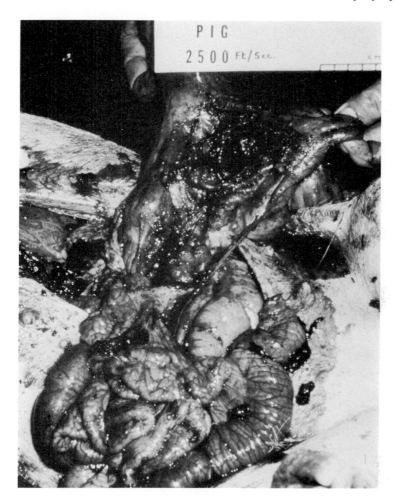

Fig. 2.20 Major destructive lesion of a whole segment of an anaesthetized pig's colon caused by standard bullet fired at 770 m/s (2500 ft/s). (Crown Copyright Reserved)

The lung itself is remarkably resistant to damage from high velocity bullets – indeed, it is true to say that lung and skin are the two tissues which are most resistant to damage from cavitation.

Low velocity bullet wounds of the liver may be very serious, particularly if they hit the vascular system, but quite commonly such bullets simply punch holes through liver tissue and, provided nothing else vital is hit, there may be very little leakage and the damage may be repairable. Direct damage from a high velocity missile is catastrophic as the liver is extremely susceptible to cavitation damage and the resultant pulping

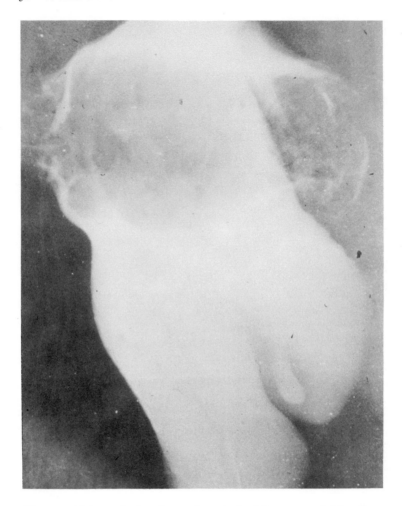

Fig. 2.21 Major cavitation changes in an isolated liver suspended in saline caused by a spherical bullet at 800 m/s (2600 ft/s). (Crown Copyright Reserved)

of liver tissue is so extensive that most cases are fatal, and the only chances of survival are usually a heroic resection of the affected lobe (Fig. 2.21). Liver and spleen are so sensitive to cavitation and shock wave that they may be damaged even when the rifle bullet passes through the chest (Fig. 2.22).

The brain is somewhat similar to the liver in being extremely susceptible to cavitation damage. Low velocity bullets, at close range, will commonly penetrate the skull but are usually arrested in the brain and it is unusual, except at point-blank range, for the bullet to come out of the other side of the head. On the other hand, a high velocity bullet

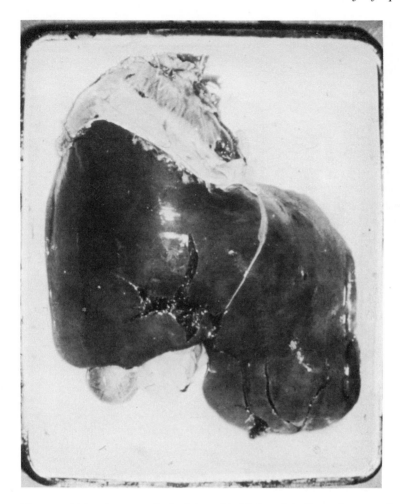

Fig. 2.22 Major damage to both right and left lobes of the liver of an anaesthetized sheep shot through the chest with a 7.62 mm rifle bullet at 100m.
(Crown Copyright Reserved)

creates a cavity in the brain and the skull is extensively fractured from within, using the brain tissue as the mechanism to effect the fracture.

This effect can be demonstrated using a human skull filled with 20 per cent gelatin to simulate brain and with a pressure transducer placed in the foramen magnum (Fig. 2.23). When a rifle bullet is fired through such a skull, pressures attained are over 400 lb/in^2. If the skull is empty, the only damage is neat entry and exit holes (Fig. 2.24).

When the skull is filled with gelatin and a bullet fired through it at the same velocity, the liquid-like medium behaves like the brain and

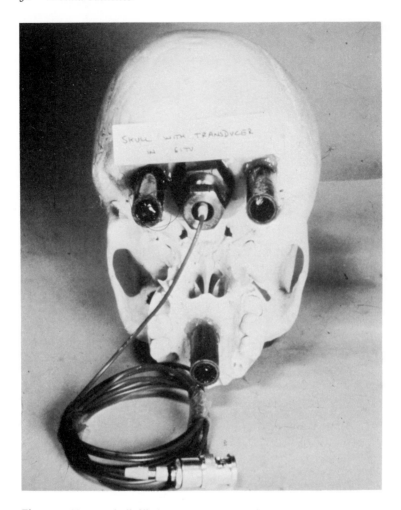

Fig. 2.23 Human skull filled with 20 per cent gelatin and with a pressure transducer placed in the foramen magnum. (Crown Copyright reserved)

allows the hydrodynamic pressure wave of cavitation to blow the skull bones apart from within, causing gross egg-shell fracturing of the skull (Figs. 2.25 and 2.26).

Large nerves are often severely damaged by the gross displacement they undergo during the cavitational process, particularly in a limb. This displacement may cause stretching of the nerve sufficient to cause a neuropraxia or axontmesis. Nerves damaged in this way show changes histologically which account for their loss of conduction and the time taken for the nerve to regenerate is usually more prolonged after such bullet injuries than from other forms of trauma.

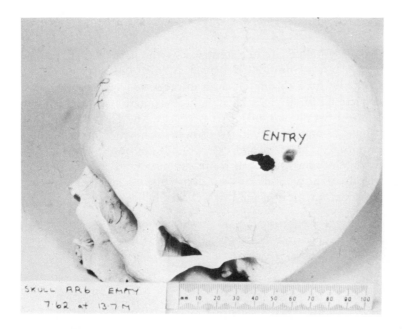

Fig. 2.24 Empty human skull showing a simple hole created by high velocity 7.62 mm bullet at 14 m range. (Crown Copyright reserved)

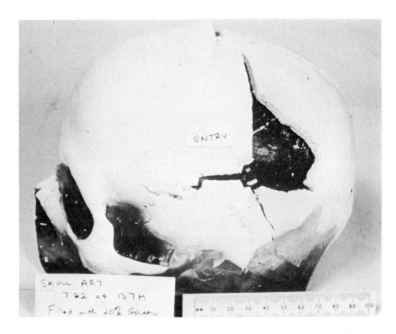

Fig. 2.25 Human skull filled with gelatin and then perforated by a high velocity 7.62 mm rifle bullet at 14 m. The major disruption of the skull by the cavitation effect is shown. (Crown Copyright Reserved)

High velocity bullets are not sterilized by the heat of their passage through the air, as is commonly believed. A bullet can be painted with bacteria and also fired through a cloth impregnated with bacteria or a cloud of bacteria. In all cases, there is gross contamination extending throughout the whole wound. This is because the passage of a high velocity bullet creates a cavity in the tissues which is at a lower pressure than that outside. The entry and exit wounds are open to this cavity, and bacteria, clothing and debris from the outside are actively sucked into the depths of the wound. This is an active process and not the passive process of contamination of the low velocity bullet.

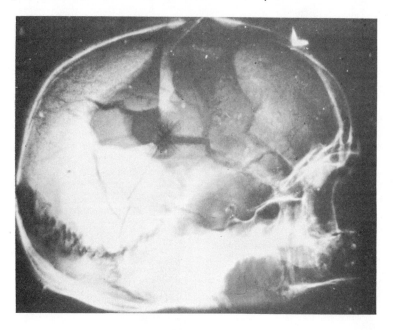

Fig. 2.26 X-ray of the skull shown in Fig. 2.25. This reveals the gross fracturing which has taken place. (Crown Copyright Reserved)

All accidental wounds are contaminated, but this is particularly true of high velocity bullet wounds as they contain a mass of pulped tissue with a gross amount of debris and bacteria. *Clostridia* spores are normally carried on the skin and clothing and most infections resulting from these organisms are autogenous. In wounds containing dead tissues, particularly muscle, the conditions are ripe for the development of clostridial myonecrosis or gas gangrene. One must remember that this is a clinical diagnosis, not a bacteriological one, and it is the one condition which above all other infections, we must strive to prevent and which was the main reason why the principles of thorough wound excision and delayed

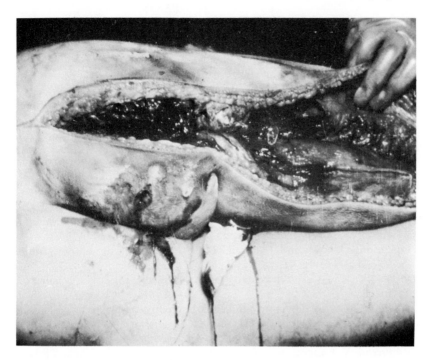

Fig. 2.27. Death from gas gangrene following high velocity bullet wounds of the buttocks and thigh. (World War II photograph by the Metal Box Company).

primary wound closure were developed and made mandatory in war surgery (Fig. 2.27).

Essential first aid, energetic resuscitation, wound excision plus delayed primary closure, early repair of arteries and the judicious use of colostomy are the essential principles which have been learned from war surgery that must be applied to missile wounds, in particular those resulting from high velocity bullets and high velocity fragments from explosive blast. These principles must be understood by all those who are concerned with the treatment of bullet-wounded patients in this country.

These principles are the distillation of the experience of many millions of casualties. They have stood the test of time and it is regrettable that they have had to be relearned the hard way in every war situation. Judicious training in the management of bullet wounds, particularly those resulting from rifle bullets, will lead to better treatment for all patients wounded by such missiles.

References and Further Reading

Berlin, R. *et al.* (1976). Local effects of assault rifle bullets in live tissues, Part I. *Acta Chirurgica Scandinavia.* Supplementum 459.

Berlin, R., *et al.* (1977). Local effects of assault rifle bullets in live tissues, Part II. *Acta Chirurgica Scandinavia.* Supplementum 477.

Black, A.N., Burns, B.D. and Zuckerman, S. (1941). An experimental study of the wounding mechanism of high velocity missiles. *British Medical Journal*, **2**, 872–74.

Callender, G.R. and French, R.W. (1935). Wound ballistics – studies in the mechanism of wound production by rifle bullets. *The Military Surgeon*, **77**, 177–201.

Coates, J.B. and Beyer, J.C. (eds) (1962). *Wound Ballistics.* Medical Department United States Army, Washington DC.

DeMuth, W.E. (1969). Bullet velocity as applied to military rifle wounding capacity. *Journal of Trauma*, **9**, 27–38.

Hopkinson, D.A.W. and Marshall, T.K. (1967). Firearm injuries. *British Journal of Surgery*, **54**, 344–53.

Horsley, V. (1894). The destructive effects of small projectiles. *Nature*, **50**, 104–8.

Krauss, M. (1957). Studies in wound ballistics: temporary cavity effects in soft tissues. *Military Medicine*, **121**, 221–31.

Owen-Smith, M.S. (1978). High velocity missile injuries. In *Current Surgical Practice* Volume 2, eds John Hadfield and Michael Hobsley, Edward Arnold. London, pp. 204–229.

Sellier, K. (1979). Effectiveness of small calibre ammunition. *Acta Chirurgica Scandinavia*, Supplement **489**, 13–26.

Skepanovic, D. (1979). The effect of shooting steel spheres at blocks of soap. *Acta Chirurgica Scandinavia.* Supplementum, **489**, 71–80.

Thoresby, F.P. (1966). Cavitation – the wounding process of the high velocity missile. *Journal of the Royal Army Medical Corps*, **112**, 89–99.

Thoresby, F.P. and Darlow, H.M. (1967). The mechanisms of primary infection of bullet wounds. *British Journal of Surgery*, **54**, 359–61.

Woodruff, C.E. (1898). The causes of the explosive effect of modern small calibre bullets. *New York Medical Journal*, **67**, 593–601.

3
Explosive blast injuries

The bomb has become an increasingly popular terrorist weapon used by extremist groups. Such bombs placed in public places can cause large numbers of casualties. Every person concerned with the care of these patients should understand how explosive devices cause injury and the principles of treatment of their wounds.

Explosives are substances which, when detonated, are very rapidly converted into large volumes of gases. When the explosion is confined by some form of bomb or shell casing, the pressure ruptures the casing imparting high velocity to the resulting fragments. The remainder of the energy then produces the blast shock wave, fire and ground shock. There are three components of the compound blast wave in air.

Positive wave

The blast wave starts with a single pulse of increased pressure lasting a few milliseconds; this layer of compressed air has an extremely sharp front less than one thousandth of an inch thick in which the pressure rises almost instantaneously to peak levels (Figs. 3.1, 3.2). It then falls rapidly to reach a minimum pressure which is less than the previous atmospheric pressure. The duration of the pulse depends on the type of explosive and the distance from the point of detonation. For trinitrotoluene (TNT) an overpressure of 100 lbf/in² (690 kPa) may be associated with a duration of 2 ms for a 25 kg charge and 10 ms for 2000 kg charge. The duration of the pulse is important, for it represents the time an object in the path of a shock wave is subjected to the pressure squeeze. The blast wave moves away from the source in the form of a sphere of compressed gas, which is expanding rapidly. The velocity of the blast shock wave in air may be as high as 3000 m/s (10 000 ft/s) but it soon falls to the speed of sound within a variable distance depending upon the amount and composition of the explosive.

The maximum pressure of the blast wave immediately adjacent to the explosive charge is extremely high. Thereafter the pressure falls off as the wave moves away from the source of the explosion. For example with TNT a 30 kg charge produces 100 lbf/in² (690 kPa) at 5 m and

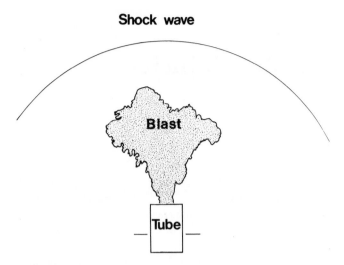

Fig. 3.1 Diagram from a high speed photograph of an explosion of a mixture of pentane and air, showing the expanding gases and the shock wave.

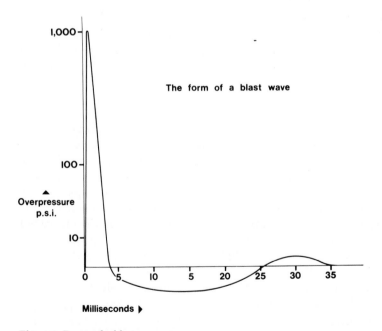

Fig. 3.2 Form of a blast wave

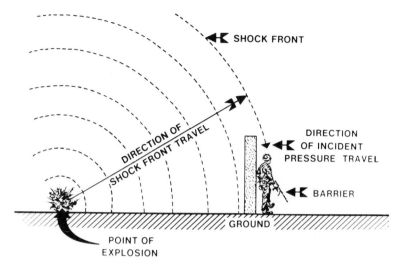

Fig. 3.3 Diagram of an explosion showing a direction of propogation of a blast wave and how the incident pressure will affect a subject sheltering behind a wall.

6 lbf/m² (41.4 kPa) at 15 m, whereas a 50 kg charge produces 200 lbf/in² (1380 kPa) at 5 m and 10 lbf/in² (69 kPa) at 15 m. These figures represent hydrostatic pressure in excess of normal atmospheric pressure.

The *incident* pressure is the pressure level at 90° to the direction of the travel of the blast shock front. Like sound waves the blast pressure waves will flow over and around an obstruction, like a wall, and affect someone sheltering behind it (Fig. 3.3). The *reflected* pressure is the rapid build up of pressure that occurs when a shock front strikes a flat surface in its line of travel, a person standing near a wall facing an explosion would be exposed to both incident and reflected pressure.

Negative phase
The negative pressure or suction component of the blast wave is much less than the positive pressure phase and can never be greater than 15 lbf/in² (103.5 kPa). It follows immediately after the positive wave but lasts about ten times as long.

Mass movement of air
The rapidly expanding gases from an explosion displace an equal volume of air and this air rushes out at very high velocity. Any surface facing an explosion will be subjected not only to excess hydrostatic pressure but also to pressure from this high velocity wind which travels immediately

Table 3.1 Blast pressure effects upon structures on open ground (DASA, 1860 (1966) from United States National Bomb Data Centre (1974)).

Pressure (lbf/in²)*	Structure of material
0.1–5	Shatter single strength glass
1–2	Crack plaster walls
	Shatter asbestos sheet
	Buckle steel sheet
	Failure of wood wall
2–3	Crack cinder block wall
	Crack concrete block wall
2–8	Crack brick wall
5–10	Shatter laminated car safety glass

* 1 lbf/in² ≈ 6.9 kPa

behind the shock front of the blast wave. This is called the *dynamic* pressure. Close to the explosion the dynamic pressure may be as great as the hydrostatic pressure of the shock front, but further from the explosion the effect falls off rapidly. The very high wind associated with blast over-pressures is emphasized by the fact that a hurricane force wind of 125 mph only exerts an overpressure of 0.25 lbf/in² (1.725 kPa), whereas an overpressure of 100 lbf/in² (690 kPa) is associated with a blast wind travelling at the velocity of Concorde (1500 mph). The effects of the blast pressure wave on structures exposed on open ground to an unconfined explosion is shown in Table 3.1. Note the low pressures that can cause severe damage which is so common in urban bomb explosions.

Explosions under water

The blast wave travels much more rapidly (1500 m/s or 5000 ft/s) and much further in water due to the greater density of the medium and its relative incompressibility. That is why blast injuries in water are more severe at a greater distance than they are in air. There is no negative phase and there is very little mass movement of water even close up to the explosion. Corresponding values for pressure are much higher in a water shock wave than in air; for example, a 250 g charge produces a peak pressure of 3000 lbf/in² (20700 kPa) at 2 m and a 100 kg charge 25 lbf/in² (172.5 kPa) at a range of 700 m.

Historical

During World War I a number of fatal casualties occurred in soldiers who had been close to the explosion of shells and mines and whose bodies showed no signs whatever of external injury. Experiments at that time and later showed that rabbits were killed if exposed at a short distance from an explosion, and that the area within which this fatal effect was caused was almost ten times as great in water than in air. The main pathology was found to be massive haemorrhage in the lungs with pulmonary and central nervous system signs. It was found that bruising and rupture of the lungs was the single gross lesion found at postmortem examination. Some animals died immediately, others after an interval and others survived; small animals like rabbits and cats died when exposed to the same blast which larger animals like dogs survived without obvious harm.

Even in 1939 there was still speculation about how pulmonary lesions were caused in air blast and in 1940 Zuckerman elucidated the matter. He carried out experiments on small animals in two ways. First, they were exposed at various distances to blast from charges of TNT placed in paper containers on the ground and in the second, the animals were exposed to blast from the explosion of charges of hydrogen and oxygen in balloons. He confirmed that there was much species variation in susceptibility, but in general the larger the animal the less severe was the damage and he noted that no lesions were observed at pressures of 5 lbf/in^2 (34.5 kPa). Small animals such as rabbits might be killed instantaneously at pressures of 50 lbf/in^2 (345 kPa) and all were killed as pressures approached 100 lbf/in^2 (690 kPa). He found that there was a range of pressure in which all animals of the same species were killed without any external signs of injury. Farther from the explosion, there was a zone of pressure in which the animals were found alive but who usually died within 24 h. His summary was that the blast of high explosives caused haemorrhagic lesions in various internal organs of the experimental animals without causing any external injury. The most conspicuous lesions were found in the lungs, where they varied from small superficial haemorrhages to haemorrhage which affected the entire substance of the lung. These lesions were also observed in other viscera and in the submucosa of the upper part of the trachea. Rupture of the eardrums was noted almost uniformly. The experiments had shown that the thoracic and abdominal lesions were due to the impact on the body wall of the pressure wave and not to any effect of the suction wave. The pulmonary lesions were thus comparable with haemorrhagic lesions which may occur as a result of severe falls or direct blows on the chest wall. Much of his work was confirmed by Krohn *et al.* (1942) and Clemedson in 1949.

After establishing the pressures that killed animals, attempts were made to find out the pressures necessary to injure those parts of the body most sensitive to blast. The ear-drums proved to be the most vulnerable. Pressures required to rupture 50 per cent of exposed drums was under 15 lbf/in^2 (103.5 kPa). The minimal pressure likely to damage the lungs was calculated to be about 50 lbf/in² (345 kPa). Benzinger (1950) protected some animals with a plaster jacket to cover the thorax and abdomen, these animals did not develop lung changes even when the tracheobronchial tree was exposed to the blast by means of a tracheostomy. Desaga (1943) showed that a unilateral pneumothorax protected the underlying collapsed lung and that damage from the blast only occurred on the lung on the opposite side.

Damage to the abdominal viscera is proportionally rare in air blast and the experiments had shown that most animals who did have abdominal injuries had been killed by the explosion. Such injuries were mainly localized to the gastro-intestinal canal especially to those parts containing gas where both haemorrhage and perforation could occur.

Spalling effects
When a shock wave travelling through one medium attempts to pass an interface with another medium of less density, there occurs at the interface a negative reflection which produces severe local tension in the first medium. As a result, the surface of the heavier medium fragments or 'spalls'; this usually occurs at an interface between a solid or liquid, which are relatively very dense, and a gas which is very much less dense. This can be demonstrated by the flakes of 'spall' that come off the inside of a rusty iron bucket when it is hit by a hammer, or when the underwater blast wave from a depth charge reaches the surface and causes a mound of broken water which is thrown into the less dense air.

Implosion effects
When an explosive produced shock wave travels in a fluid medium, or body tissues, it comes into contact with small gas bubbles, these are violently compressed with the production of very high local pressures. The bubbles 'implode' causing further shock waves and local tissue destruction.

Blast injuries in man

The concept of a blast wave is difficult and it is not easy to imagine how the body tissues react to it. It is necessary to visualize a brief but very violent blow striking the whole surface of the body on the side of the shock wave. Much of the energy of the shock wave is reflected but a proportion is transmitted through the tissues and strikes the internal organs one by one during the succeeding millisecond or so. The tissues vary in their susceptibility to this injury. The homogeneous or more solid tissues are virtually incompressible and they simply vibrate as a whole and escape serious injury. Organs containing gas such as the middle

Table 3.2 Short duration pressure effects upon unprotected persons in the open from an unconfined air explosion. (DASA, 1860 (1966) from United States National Bomb Data Centre (1974)).

Pressure (lbf/in²)★	Effect
5	Slight chance of ear-drum rupture
15	50 per cent chance of ear-drum rupture
30–50	Slight chance of lung damage
80–100	50 per cent severe lung damage
100	Slight chance of death
130–180	50 per cent chance of death
200–250	Death usually

★1 lbf/in² ≈ 6.9 kPa

ear, lungs and gastro-intestinal tract are liable to damage. This is because they are compressible and have tissue-gas interfaces. Compressibility means displacement and wherever tissues of differing densities lie side by side, this displacement may cause distortion and tearing of the tissues. Lesions are most severe at junctions between tissues, and where loose, poorly supported tissue attached to dense tissues is displaced beyond its elastic limits. Other mechanical factors such as spalling, implosion, inertial and pressure differences all interact at such sites.

Clinical experience and animal experimentation has shown that the most vulnerable organs are the ear-drums, lungs, and the gastro-intestinal tract (Table 3.2).

Auditory system
Explosive blast can damage the hearing in three ways.
1. Rupture of the tympanic membrane which occurs in human adults at pressures of about 7 lbf/in² (48.3 kPa) and even in children is usually complete by 30 lbf/in² (207 kPa).
2. Dislocation of ossicles which can take place whether or not the tympanic membrane is ruptured.
3. Damage to the inner ear. Severe deafness often occurs on exposure to explosive blast. Depending on the level of pressure much of the deafness may recover over a period of hours or days; those with irreversible inner ear damage will be permanently deaf.

Injuries to the lungs
Haemorrhages in the lung usually occur on the side turned towards the explosion. They are mainly localized to the apices and to those parts of the lung which become compressed and contused between the chest wall and the liver and the chest wall and the mediastinum. The mechanism

is probably that the lungs become compressed between the rigid spine, the inward moving thoracic wall and the rising diaphragm. The diaphragm rises violently under the ram effect of the abdominal viscera when the pressure wave compresses the abdominal wall. To this must be added the damaging effects of 'spalling' and 'implosion'. Pulmonary haemorrhage may also be explained by pressure differential gradients between the fluid and gaseous compartments of the body when struck by a pressure wave. The pressure differentials in the lung may initially precipitate pulmonary haemorrhage and then induce air emboli to enter the circulation.

In the lungs the alveolar septa are most affected. These get torn, so that the alveolar spaces join together, the lung parenchyma shears away from the tough vascular tree and the alveolar epithelium is shredded. The epithelium of the bronchioles gets stripped away from the basement membrane. The fluid-air barrier is thus breached and blood and oedema fluid escapes into the alveoli. Air is forced into the pulmonary vessels and can be demonstrated in the coronary and cerebral arteries; alveolar-venous fistulae have been demonstrated microscopically. The lung damage varies from pin-point haemorrhages in survivors up to massive intrapulmonary haemorrhages in those who die. At autopsy the pleural surface shows alternate light and dark markings. The light bands correspond to the ribs and the dark haemorrhagic bands to the intercostal spaces where the lung was not protected by bone.

Solid viscera
The solid viscera may be damaged by blast effects. The liver and spleen are the most commonly affected organs. This is not usually from the blast pressure wave but from the violent acceleration and deceleration forces caused by the blast wind blowing the subject over and hurling him against the ground or buildings.

Gastro-intestinal system
Damage to the gut is unusual in air blast but more common in underwater explosion. Gross damage and evisceration do occur in fatal cases who were very close to the centre of an explosion. When closed injuries result, they usually take the form of perforation of the air containing viscera, normally the large bowel and stomach, or multiple haemorrhages into the wall and lumen of such structures. The clinical presentation is abdominal pain and melaena, and examination reveals signs of peritonism and commonly gas under the diaphragm.

Nervous system
The neurological changes are among the most striking phenomena which follow blast. The general and focal cerebral systems do not occur

when only the head is exposed to the blast. On the other hand they are present when the trunk, but not the head, is exposed. Therefore, the cause of all cerebral symptoms must be sought in damage to the trunk. Benzinger's work strongly supports that the CNS changes are due to cerebral air embolism which originates from pulmonary damage.

Coronary artery air embolism

Benzinger proved that arterial air embolism in the coronary arteries was one of the major causes for sudden death from blast and that cerebral air embolism was the main cause for the central nervous system symptoms. After exposure to blast, air embolism in the systemic circulation is only found in the arteries and not in the veins. This makes the condition distinctly different from the syndrome of Caisson disease or decompression sickness. He showed that air enters the circulation when damage occurs to the pulmonary tissues with breaks in the interface between the air spaces and the pulmonary veins. He noted that cerebral air embolism was found at autopsy only among those animals which died immediately; cerebral focal symptoms were found among those who survived longer; all animals who were killed immediately by the explosion had air embolism of the coronary vessels whereas this was not found in the surviving animals. Arterial air embolism was induced by injecting air into the pulmonary veins of experimental animals; this caused death from coronary air embolism and as little as 1 ml of air was sufficient to cause death. He also proved that cerebral air embolism occurred in experimental animals and that the air was absorbed after about ten minutes. He demonstrated with experimental air embolism both of the coronary arteries and cerebral arteries, that the fatal effects could be completely reversed by subjecting them to positive pressure and slow decompression. He was able to save animals exposed to a previously fatal level of pressure from an explosion by placing them immediately in an atmosphere of increased pressure at 3 atm (303 kPa; 44 lbf/in²) followed by slow decompression. The animals survived a level of pressure which had previously been associated with death from coronary artery air embolism. He concluded that air embolism of the coronary arteries is by no means the only cause of death, but the theory of air embolism solves the mystery of the rapidity, uniformity and precision of death by blast.

Traumatic amputations

The mass movement of air, or windage, from an explosion is capable of causing injuries of all degrees of severity. It may simply knock people over or blow them many metres through the air to cause translational injuries. In the immediate vicinity of the explosion it may cause total disintegration of the body or atomization. Lesser levels will cause

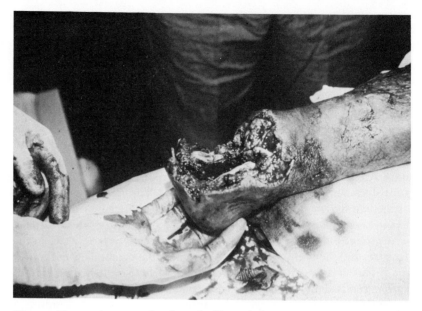

Fig. 3.4 Traumatic amputation from the blast wind.

disruption of the body into a few large or many small fragments, whereas lower levels will simply blow larger or small pieces such as a leg, a foot or toes off the body. Traumatic amputations are very common and in explosions in confined spaces we might predict that 25 per cent of the dead or severely wounded will have lost all or part of a limb (Fig. 3.4).

Treatment of explosive blast injuries

In Northern Ireland the total number of people killed by bomb explosions and bullets since 1969 approaches 2000 and nearly 20 000 have been injured. During this period the total number of recorded bomb explosions was about 6000 with over 500 killed and over 5000 wounded. Seventy of these explosions have been in England with 62 deaths out of 868 injured (Hill, 1979). Nearly 3000 people were admitted to hospital as a direct result of bullet wounds and blast injury and approximately 10 per cent of these have been admitted to the Intensive Care Unit (ICU) at the Royal Victoria Hospital, Belfast (Coppell, 1976).

The primary missiles that are sent off from the bomb casing or from the missiles such as nails, nuts and bolts, (Fig. 3.5) screws and ball bearings that are packed around home-made bombs, act as high velocity missiles and must be treated as such. That is, all penetrating wounds must be treated by thorough excision of all dead tissue, leaving the wound open and then closing them by delayed primary closure on the fourth or fifth

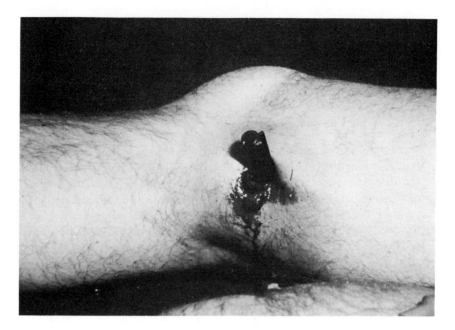

Fig. 3.5 A 6-in bolt from a home-made bomb driven through the knee joint.

day. The exceptions are wounds of the face, the dura, pleura and peritoneum which must be closed primarily. Traumatic amputations should be treated by thorough wound excision, by retaining as much viable tissue as possible and by delayed primary closure. If the wound is relatively clean, then formal flaps may be cut but should not be closed until the fourth or fifth day. The problem of the long or short or damaged stump has to be given to the limb fitting surgeon and prosthetists.

In the more unusual event of closed abdominal injuries, they should be treated according to the symptoms or signs. The most usual injury is haemorrhage into the wall of the bowel but they may also have visceral disruption. If they have signs of a perforated hollow viscus or internal bleeding then they must be explored. The following features, especially if present together, indicate the need for operation:

1. Severe unremitting abdominal pain, more especially if it increases in intensity.
2. Tenderness of the lower abdomen, particularly when there is accompanying melaena.
3. Frequent bowel evacuations with melaena, associated with difficulty in micturition or haematuria.
4. Loss of liver dullness associated with the presence of subdiaphragmatic air on a radiograph.

5. The presence of guarding or rigidity of the abdominal muscles associated with diffuse tenderness.

On account of possibly pulmonary injury from the blast wave, the administration of fluid therapy will require great caution, one must use colloid solutions and be prepared to give diuretics.

Those who complain of slight abdominal pain associated with some tenderness on palpation and slight distension, should be kept under observation for two to four days. The pain may become slightly colicky and be associated with vomiting and a desire to defaecate. Frequent bowel evacuations may even take place without developing signs of peritonitis requiring a laparotomy. There may be evidence of large bowel or rectal injury requiring surgical repair. Scrotal contusion and testicular pain are common but in themselves do not call for surgery.

Some apparently mild cases may be diagnosed wrongly as abdominal contusions and treated expectantly only to develop an intraperitoneal abscess or a faecal fistula later on. Others are less fortunate and after an interval of up to ten days show evidence of an intra-abdominal catastrophe due to an abscess bursting into the peritoneal cavity with diffuse peritonitis. In such cases the perforation is often never accurately located at laparotomy.

Further difficulty in diagnosis arises because pain and tenderness in the epigastrium may be due to a chest injury stimulating the lower intercostal nerves. The chest lesion may be a single one or in addition to an abdominal lesion. The following diagnostic guides have proved helpful in the past.

1. When clinical signs are confined to the upper abdomen the probability of a thoracic cause is considerable.
2. When the clinical signs, at first confined to the upper abdomen, spread downwards to the lower belly, an abdominal lesion is certain.
3. When the clinical signs are from the first most marked in the lower abdomen, there can be little doubt that there is intraperitoneal damage.

Gases and smoke

Explosions in confined spaces cause far worse effects than those occurring in the open. In addition to the fragment and explosive blast injuries, there will be inhalation of toxic gases and smoke so that the lungs are particularly at risk from these various threats. In the Royal Victoria Hospital, Belfast series over 650 patients were admitted following bomb explosions and of these approximately 80 were transferred to the ICU. Nineteen of these developed respiratory failure, but in only eight could the diagnosis of blast injuries of the lung be confidently made.

Blast injuries of the lungs are, therefore, surprisingly uncommon when

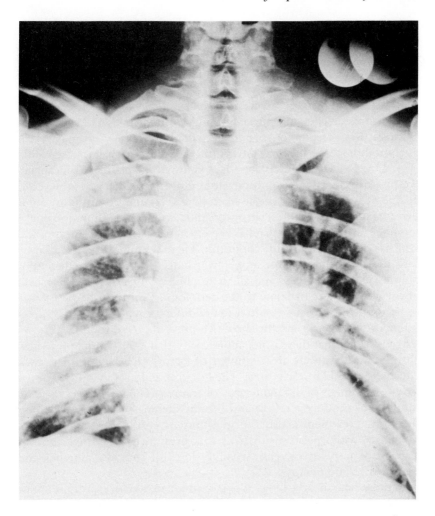

Fig. 3.6 Chest radiograph of patient suffering from blast lung. There are small opacities scattered throughout the lung fields and these represent widespread bilateral intrapulmonary haemorrhage and oedema.

it is remembered that the force of the explosion is sufficient to cause traumatic amputations or disintegration of the body at close range. Lung damage can arise from the primary blast effect and also from the patient being thrown against a solid object in the environment by the force of the explosion.

Patients with primary blast injuries of the lungs usually present with signs of anoxia. They may have dyspnoea of sudden onset, haemoptysis, cyanosis, moist crepitations in both lung fields and chest x-ray may reveal pneumothoraces or bilateral intrapulmonary haemorrhage and oedema (Fig. 3.6). External injuries may be extensive or relatively superficial. Respiratory failure commonly develops after 12–36 h delay and this could be due to a combination of the blast effects, fat embolism syndrome if there are multiple fractures, iatrogenic fluid overload or aspiration pneumonia. The terminology that has been used to describe this pathological state has caused considerable confusion. There is a multiplicity of phrases such as 'shock lung', 'blast lung', 'wet lung' 'stiff lung', 'high putput pulmonary insufficiency' and all these phrases just describe one aspect of the clinical state or relate to the aetiology. Probably the best name to be applied to the end result of many different types of insult is 'post-traumatic pulmonary insufficiency' (Moore *et al.*, 1969) for this acknowledges the fact that there is no single entity that is responsible for these changes but that there are a number of factors each having their own effect and related to each other. The lung can only respond in a limited way to a number of different types of trauma. The total effect of these insults is to produce a severe and life-threatening impairment of lung function. Treatment consists of intermittent positive pressure ventilation, often with a positive end expiratory pressure (PEEP), high concentrations of inspired oxygen, massive doses of steriods, diuretics and vigorous physiotherapy.

In those who die, the lungs at postmortem are like liver in appearance and are heavy, haemorrhagic and oedematous. The rib markings can often be seen, with multiple punctate haemorrhages occurring along the intercostal spaces. Lacerations, if present, are often found along these lines.

Awareness of blast injuries

The severity of a blast lesion appears to be in direct relationship to the distance from the explosion. Those near the centre of a large explosion will usually be killed instantly while those at a greater distance will survive. The further away a person is from an explosion the less likely is the chance of injury. Patients with blast injuries are commonly apprehensive and tremulous, and may be wrongly diagnosed as having battle neurosis. They may present no external evidence of injury and may unwittingly be returned to their units or treated as walking wounded until shock, dyspnoea or other features call attention to the gravity of their condition. Patients who have sustained other more obvious injuries such as compound fractures may indeed receive general anaesthesia or rapid intravenous transfusion of crystalloids with dire consequences if a condition like the blast lung is overlooked. Other inhalation injuries may co-exist and indeed may readily occur under the conditions in which explosive blast damage has been sustained. A person who is clinically shocked, who has been near an explosive device but who has no apparent wounds or contusions may be suffering from blast injury and a high index of suspicion under these circumstances must be maintained.

References and Further Reading

Benzinger, T. (1950). *German Aviation Medicine in World War II.* Vol. 2, United States Department of the Air Force, Ch. 14.

Cameron, G.R., Short, R.H.D. and Wakeley, C.P.G. (1941). Pathological changes produced in animals by depth charges. *British Journal of Surgery*, **30,** 49–64.

Cameron, G.R., Short, R.H.D. and Wakeley, C.P.G. (1942). Abdominal injuries due to underwater explosions. *British Journal of Surgery*, **31,** 51–66.

Candole, C.A. de (1967). Blast injury. *Canadian Medical Association Journal*, **96,** 207–14.

Clemedson, C.J. (1949). An experimental study of air blast injuries. *Acta Physiologica Scandinavica*, **18,** Supplementum 61.

Coppell, D.L. (1976). Blast injuries of the lung. *British Journal of Surgery*, **63,** 735–37.

Desaga, H. (1943). Quoted by Benzinger (1950).

Hooker, D.K. (1924). Physiological effects of air concussion. *American Journal of Physiology*, **67,** 219–74.

Hill, J. (1979). Blast injury with particular reference to recent terrorist bombing incidents. *Annals of the Royal College of Surgeons of England*, **61,** 4–11.

Krohn, P.L., Whitteridge, D. and Zuckerman, S. (1942). Physiological effects of blast. *Lancet*, **1,** 252–58.

Mathew, W.E. (1917). Notes of the effects produced by a submarine mine explosion. *Journal of the Royal Naval Medical Service*, **3,** 108–9.

Moore, F.D. *et al.* (1969). *Post-traumatic Pulmonary Insufficiency.* W.B. Saunders and Company Philadelphia.

Owen-Smith, M.S. (1979). Explosive blast injury. *Journal of the Royal Army Medical Corps*, **125,** 4–16.

Rawlins, J.S.P. (1978). Physical and pathophysiological effects of blast. *Injury*, **9,** 313–20.

United States National Bomb Data Center (1974). *General Information Bulletin*, Bulletin No. 74–9.

Waterworth, T.A. and Carr, M.J.T. (1973). An analysis of the PM findings in the 21 victims of the Birmingham pub bombings. *Injury*, **7,** 89–95.

Williams, E.R.P. (1941). Blast effects in warfare. *British Journal of Surgery*, **30,** 38–49.

Zuckerman, S. (1940). Experimental study of blast injuries to the lungs. *Lancet*, **ii,** 219–24.

Zuckerman, S. (1941). Discussion on the problems of blast injuries. *Proceedings of the Royal Society of Medicine*, **34,** 171–88.

Part 2
Principles of Treatment

4

Primary treatment
of the wounded

Casualty sorting – triage

The importance of sorting casualties has been emphasized in two World Wars and the term 'triage' has been applied to the sorting of military casualties since that time. Triager is a French word which means to sort into groups according to quality. The concept of casualty sorting or triage has also been extended to civilian disaster situations with considerable benefit and its use is now generally accepted. Triage can take place anywhere on the line of evacuation of the casualty from the point of injury to the hospital where definitive treatment is done.

The aims of triage are to sort out a mass of casualties in a logical fashion based on the severity of injury, the need for treatment, the possibilities of good quality survival and the surgical and medical care available for their treatment. It involves the establishment of priorities for treatment and evacuation; essentially the decisions that have to be made concern the need for resuscitation, the need for emergency life-saving or limb-saving surgery and, finally, the futility of surgery because of the intrinsic lethality of the wound.

Successful triage depends upon taking into account all the factors which affect the casualties. The number and nature of the wounded, their condition, the facilities and personnel available to treat them and, finally, the line of evacuation and the duration of such travel.

Effective triage at the site of the disaster leads to the most logical and orderly evacuation of the wounded, the most efficient use of stretchers, ambulances and other transport and the optimum use of medical and surgical expertise. Time is usually at a premium in such a situation so the system of casualty sorting must be simple. Rapid assessment of casualties can be taught, not only to doctors but to nurses, ambulance, police and fire brigade staff and first-aiders. It should, therefore, be possible to implement triage at any point on the line of evacuation.

No task in the medical service requires skilled judgement more than the sorting of casualties. When a number of seriously injured casualties arrive within a short space of time, it is important that the most experienced person in management of such cases should be designated the triage or sorting doctor. He must exercise sound surgical judgement when deciding which patients need immediate resuscitation, which patients require resuscitation and immediate surgery as part of the resuscitation process and those which tolerate some delay before receiving surgical attention.

In any group of people who are injured, for example, a large number who may be involved as a result of a bomb explosion, there exists subgroups who can be divided in the following way:

Group A. Those whose injuries are so slight that they can be managed by self-help. They must be rapidly segregated from the other groups and not allowed to interfere with the management of the more severely wounded.

Group B. Those whose wounds require medical evaluation and care but which are so slight that they can be managed by simple treatment and dressings available in the casualty or emergency department of the hospital. These casualties can be readily segregated from the rest and may be sent a considerable distance to other hospitals which are not over-taxed by the number of severely injured casualties.

Group C. Those whose injuries demand surgical attention and operation. These are further categorized into Priorities 1–3.

Group D. Those who are dead or who have such severe wounds that death is inevitable.

It is those patients in Group C who requires urgent resuscitation and/or surgery that most care will be concentrated upon. Casualties are sorted into three priorities basically as follows:

Priority 1. Cases requiring resuscitation and urgent surgery. The majority of preventable deaths that occur as a result of missile wounds are from asphyxia and haemorrhage. Therefore any wounded patients suffering from these two conditions must be treated and evacuated as a matter of urgency. Asphyxia can be from respiratory obstruction from mechanical causes, sucking chest wounds, tension pneumothorax and in some maxillofacial wounds. Shock is caused by major external haemorrhage, major internal haemorrhage, visceral injuries or evisceration, cardiopericardial injuries, massive muscle damage, particularly when associated with major fractures, multiple wounds and severe burns of over 20 per cent. As shock will occur in many of these injuries it is imperative to commence treatment in anticipation of its development.

Priority 2. These are cases who require early surgery, possibly associated with resuscitation. Examples are: visceral injuries, including perforation of the gastrointestinal tract, wounds of the biliary and pancreatic system, wounds of the genito-urinary system, thoracic wounds without asphyxia, vascular injuries requiring repair, closed cerebral injuries with increasing loss of consciousness.

Priority 3. Cases requiring less urgent surgery. Provided that there is no immediate risk of life or limb and that there is no need for immediate resuscitation, this group of patients may well be fit to travel some considerable distance after receiving essential first aid. Examples are: spinal injuries requiring decompression, soft tissue injuries of less than major degree, lesser fractures and dislocations, eye injuries and maxillofacial injuries without aphyxia, burns of under 20 per cent. Such patients may well be able to travel for a number of hours to distant hospitals when circumstances dictate this.

This system works very well in practice. The distinction between Priority 1 and Priority 2 is not always clear but these are always the patients who will be evacuated as rapidly as possible to the nearest surgical facility. All the other wounded can be moved at a slightly less urgent pace.

Mass casualties
When a situation of casualty overload exists, the number of casualties who require urgent or early treatment is too much for the surgical capability available. Such a situation may obviously exist in both conventional war or nuclear war, but it also exists at a local level whenever a relatively large number of casualties occur and under these circumstances conventional treatment priorities must be abandoned. Whenever possible casualties should be diverted to other hospitals so that only the nearest and most suitably equipped and established hospitals deal with the Priority 1 and Priority 2 cases. When even this system is overloaded then a new system of casualty sorting has to be implemented until such time as order is obtained out of chaos and that those who are in need of urgent treatment to save their life obtain it. The problem of treating large numbers of wounded with locally limited resources requires the exercize of considerable judgement and expertise. Patients must be classified, not only as to type and severity of injury but an assesssment must also be made of the likelihood of good quality survival. A rather different system of priorities for treatment and evacuation must be established in order to assure medical care for the greatest benefit of the largest number. It is not possible to lay down a set of rules which will apply in all circumstances because there are so many variable factors but it is usual to classify patients according to their need for medical care and also their chance of survival. The following classification gives examples in each group and forms a framework into which details can be inserted. In a mass casualty situation the following classification has been implemented by the NATO Armed Services. Similar classifications are in use, or being developed in most regions of the country.

T1 Immediate treatment
T2 Delayed treatment
T3 Minimal treatment
T4 Expectant treatment

T1 Immediate treatment. This group includes those patients who require some form of first-aid surgery necessary to save life or limb. The procedure should not be time-consuming and should concern only those patients in whom the chances of good quality survival are high. About twenty minutes is the time scale that is suggested for each operation. Examples are: respiratory obstruction from whatever cause, accessible severe haemorrhage and first aid amputations.

T2 Delayed treatment. This group comprises those who are fit for evacuation and who need time-consuming surgical treatment but whose lives will not be unduly endangered by some delay. The amount of this delay will often be critical but its effect can be minimized by the use of antibiotics, intravenous fluids, nasogastric suction, catheterization, analgesics and skilled first aid. Examples are: fractures of major bones, large muscle wounds, intra-abdominal injury, thoracic injury, head or spinal injuries and burns of up to 30 per cent.

T3 Minimal treatment. This constitutes a very large group for it includes all those with a relatively minor injury who can be dealt with effectively when first seen by a doctor or other medical attendant. Thereafter they can largely care for themselves or be helped by relatively untrained personnel. Examples of this are: small lacerations or abrasions, closed fractures of small bones, small burns of less than 10 per cent body surface area.

T4 Expectant treatment. This group comprises those patients who have serious, and often multiple, injuries whose treatment will be difficult, time-consuming and complicated and which make enormous demands on medical manpower and supplies. Under the best conditions their prognosis is poor. They should not be allowed to enter and clog the evacuation route, but should receive appropriate supportive treatment locally. The extent of treatment will depend upon available supplies and manpower. These patients should not be abandoned but efforts should be made to make them comfortable and the possibility of survival with even the most extensive injuries must always be kept in mind. Examples are: severe head or spinal injuries, severe multiple injuries, burns of more than 30 per cent. This presupposes that those who are dead have been certified as such as they, therefore, have no priority for treatment allocated. It is important that this recognition and marking of the dead should be performed by the sorting medical personnel in order that time and effort is not wasted upon them.

It is essential to recognize that casualty sorting is a dynamic and not a static process. Many factors affect a decision and significant alteration in one of these factors may allow the patient to be placed into a new category. The total situation must be kept under review all the time during treatment or evacuation.

Good records are essential and it is important, in a mass casualty situation, to have tie-on medical record cards for the injured which, ideally, includes a unique number and details of type and site of injury, their priority for evacuation and treatment.

First-aid

The essentials of first aid are to prevent death and avoid further injury. Most deaths that occur after injury from bullet wounds and explosive blast are due to loss of cardiorespiratory function and haemorrhage. If these two problems can be controlled then there is an excellent chance that the patient will survive until he reaches hospital.

Airway

Respiratory obstruction is an emergency of the utmost importance. Speed in relieving respiratory obstruction and maintaining an adequate flow of air to the lungs is essential and cannot be emphasized too strongly. In an unconscious patient, when respiratory obstruction is present, an efficient airway must be maintained by clearing the mouth and pharynx, by extending the neck and by turning the patient into the semiprone or 'coma' position. If the airway cannot be maintained in this fashion then an oropharyngeal airway should be inserted. If this is not effective then it would be necessary to pass an endotracheal tube and in an emergency any rubber or other flexible tubing of suitable calibre can be used for this purpose.

Respiratory obstruction can result from a number of different causes.
1. The aspiration of blood, foreign bodies or vomitus.
2. Obstruction from the tongue. This can usually be controlled by extension of the neck and placing the patient in the semiprone position. An oropharyngeal airway will maintain an adequate airway under these circumstances.
3. Laryngeal obstruction from foreign bodies such as loose teeth or pieces of dentures, food and blood clot. The obstructing foreign bodies can usually be removed manually.
4. Oedema of the pharynx or larynx caused by inhalation burns. Under these circumstances an endotracheal tube will be necessary.
5. Tracheostomy should not be necessary as a first-aid measure in most circumstances. Probably the only recognized indication is direct

laryngeal injury when the use of an endotracheal tube would be hazardous.

Breathing

When breathing stops as a result of primary injury, it is vital to restore ventilation immediately. Artifical respiration should be continued until normal breathing returns. There are a number of methods of artificial respiration that can be used in the first-aid situation. The exhaled air method (EAR) is the easiest to use in most circumstances. This method has been shown to be superior to any of the manual methods of artificial respiration. It can be given by two methods – the mouth-to-mouth method and the mouth-to-nose method. A third alternative is mouth-to-mouth but using a specially designed oropharyngeal airway with a mouthpiece for the use of the rescuer. There are a few occasions when manual methods of artificial respiration would be required. For example, a casualty with severe face or jaw injuries or when there is a contaminated atmosphere and protective masks are in use. Under these circumstances the Silvester method of chest pressure and arm lift technique with the patient in the supine position is used.

Circulation

If the heart has stopped as an indirect result of the injury then external cardiac compression must be initiated. This will often have to be carried out in conjunction with artificial respiration.

Accessible haemorrhage

Internal haemorrhage from a penetrating wound cannot be controlled without surgery and, therefore, these patients have a top priority for evacuation. External haemorrhage can usually be controlled by direct pressure. A dressing or any available material can be packed closely and carefully into a wound and this will usually stop the bleeding. If a blood vessel can be seen in the depths of the wound and it is continuing to bleed then direct control may be obtained either manually or with artery forceps if they are available. Blind clamping must never be attempted. Pressure applied to the pressure points over an artery may be of use in reducing haemorrhage until control can be attained.

A tourniquet is rarely required, its application can save life but it also threatens the limb unless it is correctly applied for the right reasons and removed when facilities are available for adequate control of the bleeding. In general it should only be applied as a last resort and accepting the risks that go with its application. Together with the control of accessible haemorrhage comes the problem of replacing fluid loss. In a first-aid situation if equipment is available and evacuation is delayed then an intravenous drip should be set up using Hartmann's solution initially. Blood can be taken for grouping and cross-matching to be sent with, or ahead of, the patient to hospital.

Chest wounds

Penetrating chest wounds may have a serious effect on respiration for they can damage the heart and mediastinal structures or the lungs. They always create a pneumothorax which may be small or large but is commonly closed, and there is always some degree of haemothorax. A penetrating wound of the chest may create a hole which stays open. This creates an open pneumothorax in which air passing in and out of the pleural cavity, and bubbling through the blood coming from the wound, creates a characteristic sucking or blowing noise. Such a wound is known traditionally as a sucking wound of the chest and the problem is that there may be grave physiological changes which can result in rapid death unless they are treated. The first-aid treatment is to seal the wound to minimize the physiological changes and to allow the remaining, undamaged, lung to function better. The wound should be sealed using an airtight dressing. This can be improvized and made from a wet bulky dressing that is securely fixed into place or, if available, a more effective seal can be obtained using Vaseline gauze next to the wound, covered with a further dressing.

A tension pneumothorax may result from either penetrating chest wounds or from explosive blast injury. It may also occur when a sucking chest wound has been sealed by an occlusive dressing and this should be anticipated. Tension pneumothorax is an acute emergency and must be treated by insertion of a large bore chest tube connected to a one-way valve of the Heimlich type. The tube should be inserted in the second intercostal space in the mid-clavicular line. If a tube is not available any large bore needle will relieve the tension pneumothorax, in these circumstances a flutter valve can be improvized from the finger of a rubber glove.

A flail segment of the chest wall may result from closed injuries in which the number of ribs broken result in an unstable segment of chest wall and consequent paradoxical respiration. The physiological changes from this injury are minimized by firmly strapping the affected segment of chest wall and by careful positioning of the patient so that the damaged segment is against the ground, bed or stretcher. It is stressed that these problems come more from the bruised, poorly functioning lung rather than the paradoxical movement. Transportation of all patients with chest injuries should be with the uninjured side uppermost to allow optimal ventilation of the good lung.

Dressings and splints

The majority of fractures do not need complicated splintage when evacuation is going to be over a short space of time. Inflatable splints are excellent for this purpose as they are quick to apply, do not interfere with x-rays and give adequate immobilization. The upper limbs may be splinted in a sling or by using the patient's clothing. The leg may be splinted effectively, using any materials that are available, to the good leg. If there is any delay in evacuation or the duration of such evacuation will be prolonged then it is of great importance to immobilize compound fractures of the femur and fractures around the knee joint and the best method for such injuries is still the Thomas's splint.

It is emphasized that most injuries will not be made much worse by leaving them alone or carrying out the minimum of first-aid dressing and splintage. The most important function of first-aid is the life-saving aspect and to stress these once again they are: attention to the airway, including the care of the unconscious patient; to close the sucking wound of the chest and to stop accessible haemorrhage.

Evacuation

In all forms of trauma, including penetrating wounds, the patient's condition should be stabilized before being evacuated. Skilled first-aid at the site of injury should allow this stability to be achieved in the vast majority of cases. A moving ambulance or helicopter is no place to attemp to put up a drip, to insert an endotracheal tube or to give intravenous injections. One must remember that the maintenance of resuscitation that has already commenced may be made much more difficult during evacuation because of the relative positions of the patient and operator and the movement of the vehicle.

Research investigations (Snook, 1972) have shown that due to defects in the interior lay-out, the suspension system, lighting and sound-proofing it was found that most ambulances impose physiological stresses upon the patient that might well cause a deterioration related to movement and vibration in the vehicle. Such stresses are made worse when travelling fast and when gravitational forces are thereby increased. When attention is paid to improved design of ambulances and where movement is made carefully and gently then the stresses are so reduced that even very seriously ill patients who are transferred between hospitals have very little ill-effects from their journey. The traditional reporting of the media that 'the patient was rushed to hospital' is one which is no longer acceptable with the seriously ill. In war-time and in difficult terrain, speed of evacuation is still essential but this means an efficient and smooth means of communication not sheer physical speed. In the urban environment if speed is required on an ambulance driver it is on the journey to the accident – speed in getting to the patient, skill in attending to his injuries and smoothness in transporting him to hospital. An ambulance is, at present, a compromise between its various functions, conflicting requirements of design affects the suspension of the vehicle with the result that cornering and comfort of ride fall measurably short of that which might be achieved if the complete vehicle was purpose-built. A vehicle must therefore be driven so that the comfort and condition of the patient is affected as little as possible so that the ambulance attendant may continue his life-support tasks or observation of the patient.

Only a very small number of patients die from remediable causes following missile wounds. Provided that skilled first-aid has been given to maintain the airway and ventilation, to close the sucking wound of the chest and to stop accessible haemorrhage then there is very little else that can be done until the patient reaches a surgical facility where operation can be performed. The major cause of exsanguination and death is likely to be a penetrating wound of the abdomen or central chest in which access to control the haemorrhage is not possible. A rapid infusion of Hartman's solution may buy some precious time and it is possible to apply antigravity suits to the lower half of the body. These were first developed for pilots of high performance aircraft and spacemen, but these suits have been adopted for use in some part of the United States and are known as Military Anti-Shock Trousers (MAST). It consists of a one-piece, double layered, elasticated material suit which covers the lower limbs and abdomen. This pneumatic garment can be pumped up so that pressure is raised within the suit and applied to the lower half of the body. It has proved effective in the control of haemorrhagic shock particularly when evacuation is delayed such as in rural areas. When inflated they can create a rapid autotransfusion of approximately one litre of blood with the additional advantages of control of lower extremity and abdominal bleeding and the stabilization of fractures. They have their enthusiastic advocates but a lot depends on the number of times they are likely to be used, the type of injuries met with in a particular locality and the pattern of evacuation times before electing to adopt their use.

During evacuation, communication by two-way radio is most useful for then the receiving hospital knows when a seriously injured casualty is on the way and appropriate reception and treatment of the casualty can be organized.

Assessment and resuscitation

In most hospitals there is very little opportunity for young doctors to gain much experience in the assessment and management of severly injured patients, and even less with those injured by bullet or blast. Unless severe injuries are centralized in large Accident and Emergency Departments it is unlikely that much expertise can be gained, at least in the training grades.

Regrettably the great pool of knowledge of severe trauma is associated primarily with war. It is only in war-time that the whole medical effort of the country is devoted with single minded purpose to give the soldier wounded in battle the best possible treatment. In that effort each surgeon is prepared to sink his individuality, to take the task allotted to him, to learn from others and share his knowledge freely. The whole sum of knowledge gained from that experience is employed and all obstacles are overcome to make it available to the injured patient in a way that it rarely is outside war.

Team work in major trauma is vital to the quality of care and the prognosis of the patient. Practice makes perfect and there is little doubt that as a team builds up experience the results improve. The chain of treatment from the point of wounding to definitive surgical treatment are all vital links in the effort. Skilled first-aid and rapid evacuation should keep a wounded but living person alive until the Accident Department is reached. Preliminary warning might well be given by radio communication from the site of injury or the ambulance in time to assemble the team.

With experience, assessment of the severely wounded patient is a rapid and almost instinctive reaction. The preservation of life relies on the application of priorities in treatment; most patients who die from remediable causes do so from asphyxia or shock.

Asphyxia comes from an obstruction to the airway or from physiological stresses imposed by a sucking wound of the chest, pneumothorax, haemothorax or haemopericardium.

Shock comes from blood loss either externally and remediable, or internally and only controllable by operation. Advanced warning of the cause of injury may anticipate the severity of wounding and allow some preparation to be made.

Airway

The first priority in treatment must be to the airway and to respiration. The airway must be cleared by removing debris and foreign bodies manually from the mouth and oropharynx, suction must be used where necessary. If the patient is unconscious or if there are fractures of the facial skeleton or major lacerations, an oropharyngeal airway must be inserted and the neck extended to allow free passage of air down to the larynx and trachea. If control is still not obtained an endotracheal tube must be passed and artificial ventilation commenced. Deeply unconscious patients may usually be intubated easily, but some may be restless, irritable, unco-operative and hypoxic. Intubation under these circumstances usually requires sedation and 5–10 mg of diazepam intravenously will allow rapid intubation without struggling and without compromising the patient's hypoxic condition.

Tracheostomy should usually be done electively and the only specific indication for emergency tracheostomy in missile wounds is direct laryngeal injury. In a desperate emergency cricothyroidotomy (coniotomy) has shown considerable advantages over tracheostomy and might well be the treatment of choice in the future.

Respiratory embarrassment

Any cause for respiratory difficulties must be found and treated. Clinical examination will reveal a sucking wound of the chest, pneumothorax, tension pneumothorax, haemothorax or a flail segment of the chest.

The sucking wound must be treated by the application of an air-tight seal dressing, best made with a piece of tulle gras or plastic sheeting covered with a bulky dressing firmly taped into place. The patient should then be positioned with the uninjured side uppermost, so allowing maximum ventillation of the undamaged lung.

An intercostal catheter should be inserted into the second space anteriorly for a pneumothorax or tension pneumothorax and a Heimlich one-way valve attached. An underwater seal can replace the valve later on.

A haemothorax should be drained by a wide-bore chest catheter inserted in the eighth or ninth intercostal space in the mid-axillary line, this should be connected to an underwater seal as soon as possible as a Heimlich valve may block with blood. This can be a life-saving measure and must be done on clinical grounds rather than awaiting confirmation of a large haemothorax by radiography.

In the rare case of a survivor with a penetrating missile wound of the heart and constrictive haemopericardium, immediate treatment is to aspirate the pericardium repeatedly until emergency thoracotomy is possible.

Shock

In missile wounds shock usually comes from acute blood loss; neurogenic shock is surprisingly unimportant in major missile wounds. The clinical signs of blood loss may be obvious, or may be inferred from experience of the type of wound.

Severe bleeding can usually be stopped by packing, provided that the source is accessible. Any material can be used in an emergency but it must be packed into the wound carefully using small quantities first, then a more bulky dressing and finally a firm elasticated bandage to apply even pressure to effect haemostasis. Finger pressure or direct application of artery forceps may occasionally be required. Once a wound has been packed and bleeding arrested then it should not be disturbed until the patient has been resuscitated and is in the operating theatre with blood available and the surgical team ready to secure bleeding by rapid access to the major blood vessels of the affected part.

Severe internal bleeding requires urgent operation as part of the resuscitation process, such patients have a high priority for surgery when a number of wounded patients are seen together.

Fluid replacement

The type of fluid for replacement is less important than the speed of re-action and getting the infusion running rapidly into the patient. A litre *now* is worth several litres in a few hours time. It is good planning to have such initial intravenous fluid ready prepared, with drip sets and needles, for immediate insertion into the veins. In massive injury with obviously gross blood loss several wide bore intravenous lines should be established and fluid pumped in rapidly to prevent the disastrous sequelae of exsanguination. One line may be placed as a CVP monitor and the bladder should be catheterized. Balanced electrolyte solution such as Hartmann's or Ringer lactate is an excellent electrolyte fluid to use for resuscitation in acute trauma.

Blood should first be taken for grouping and cross-matching and then fluid replacement can begin with 2000 ml of Hartmann's in 15–30 minutes together with 500 ml of Dextran 70 (mol. wt. = 70 000). The response must be monitored clinically, by observing urinary output and the central venous pressure. It is usual for a patient to require whole blood during the first 10 min of resuscitation but in moribund, exsanguinated patients Group O blood must be given rapidly together with the Hartmann's, as the threat of death outweighs the potential morbidity from transfusion reaction. Type-specific whole blood should be available after 10 min and cross-matched blood in 30–40 min. When blood is used for major trauma cases a microfilter should be inserted into the drip set. The standard filters take out particles larger than 17 μm whereas the microfilters prevent the passage of particles larger than 10 μm. These filters do not significantly restrict the rate of tranfusion but should not be used when fresh blood and platelets are being given.

Large quantities of blood and Hartmann's may be required. Every fourth pack of blood should be supplemented with one bottle of plasma, one ampoule of sodium bicarbonate (44.3 mE) and one ampoule of calcium chloride (10 g).

The object of resuscitation is to restore circulating blood volume and intracellular fluid, to restore normal blood flow and tissue perfusion, to attain a urine output of 25–50 ml/h and all this without overloading the lungs and adding to post-traumatic pulmonary insufficiency.

A rapid response to resuscitation allows surgery to be performed at the optimum time according to the priority for treatment. Failure to respond usually occurs as a result of internal bleeding from the trunk and urgent operation to secure the bleeding source is part of the resuscitation process. Once bleeding has been controlled the fluid and blood replacement will improve the patient's condition.

Rapid control of the airway, the insertion of chest tubes, stopping bleeding by packing or operation and the restitution of blood volume by early and rapid infusion of Hartmann's solution and blood are the corner stones of successful treatment in major penetrating missile wounds.

References and Further Reading

Snook, R. (1942). Medical aspects of ambulance design. *British Medical Journal*, **3**, 574–8.

5
Wounds of soft tissue

Technique of wound excision

Clothing, dressings and splints are carefully removed. A sterile gauze pad is held over the wound whilst the skin over a large surrounding area and the whole circumference of the limb is cleansed with detergent, shaved, dried and then painted with an antiseptic such as Hibitane in spirit, or Betadine. In the case of multiple wounds the posterior aspect of body and limbs should be dealt with before those on the anterior aspect in order to minimize turning the patient.

Incision
Skin is very resistant to damage and is remarkably viable; it should be treated conservatively. Only skin that is grossly pulped should be excised and this means that usually not more than 1–2 mm of the skin edge should ever be removed. In order to get to the depths of the wound, the skin should be incised generously. In the limbs the incision should be made along the long axis but not over subcutaneous bones, and at flexion creases it should deviate in the usual way. The subcutaneous fat has a poor blood supply and is liable to be heavily contaminated. This layer and the shredded fascia about the wound should be excised generously.

Retraction and fasciotomy
The deep fascia must be incised along the length of the incision. This essential step allows wide and deep retraction without tension thus exposing the depths of the wound. It may be necessary to add transverse cuts to the deep fascia at either end of the wound to improve access. Undamaged fascial compartments may need decompression to avoid ischaemic changes when the muscles swell in response to trauma.

Excision of dead muscle
This must be thorough, as dead muscle is the ideal medium for the development of clostridial sepsis leading to gas gangrene. The permanent

track of the missile is the one that you can see, but this track is surrounded by dead muscle and this must be excised **always**. All muscle which is not healthy and red, which does not contract or bleed when cut, must be excised until healthy contractile, bleeding muscle is reached. The technique of this procedure is simply to pick up lumps of dead muscle with forceps, pinch them and if they do not contract excise them using scissors.

Foreign bodies

The edges of the wound should be retracted and blood clot, dirt, debris and missiles are then removed from the sides and depths of the wound. Gentle and copious irrigation with saline must be used to wash out the residual debris and blood clot. Explore the wound with the finger to identify foreign bodies, unexpected extensions of the wound and remember **not** to open up fresh planes in healthy tissue. Do **not** explore for metallic fragments for a long time; instead clinical and radiological localization may indicate that they can be approached by a separate incision through fascial planes rather than by cutting through healthy muscle.

Decompression

The widely opened deep fascia which has been freely incised is left open to allow postoperative oedematous and congested tissue to swell without tension and so avoid interference with the blood supply.

Limitation of closure

All wounds should be left widely open without suture of the skin or deep structures with the following exceptions:

Face and neck
These wounds may be closed primarily after primary wound excision.

Soft tissues of chest wall
These must be excised but healthy muscle must be closed over a sucking chest wound in order to make an air-tight closure, but the skin is left open.

Head injuries
The dura is closed, directly or by temporalis fascia graft and the skin is closed by rotating flaps to provide cover.

Hand injuries
Some injuries may be closed primarily, but usually these are left open for delayed closure, tendon and nerve must be covered. Preserve **all** viable tissue as this simplifies reconstructive procedure.

Joints
The synovial membrane should be closed, if this is not possible then the capsule should be closed. If it cannot be closed then the chances are that the joint is irretrievably damaged and may be left open with the joint in the position of function.

Blood vessels
Those that have been repaired should be covered by viable muscle.

Dressings
Dry gauze is laid across the open wound and then this is covered by a bulky, fluffed up, absorbant dressing. The dressing must never be packed into the wound as this acts as a plug and for the same reason tulle gras should not be used. The whole dressing is held in place by plaster applied longitudinally. Strapping must **never** go right around a limb.

Immobilization
In all cases where there is an extensive soft tissue wound, even in the absence of a fracture, the limb as a whole is immobilized. This can be effected by splints, well padded plasters which must be split down to skin at the time the plaster is applied, or by POP slabs.

Delayed primary closure

Provided that the dead tissues of the wound resulting from high velocity missile injuries have been thoroughly excised there should be no necessity for further inspection of the wound until the time comes for closure. If there is a specific indication, such as excessive pain, oedema, or if there are signs of infection then it may be necessary to inspect the wound in the theatre under a general anaesthetic. This is usually an indication that wound excision has been incomplete and a further excision of dead tissue is necessary.

When initial wound excision has been adequate the open missile wound will continue to ooze blood and serum for two days. The wound is sealed by coagulated serum on the the third day and early granulations appear over the surface of the fibrinous coagulum between the third and the fifth day. This period from the third to the fifth day forms the optimum time for delayed closure of such wounds. This time was found empirically but this optimum time for closure has been proven experimentally and by controlled trials to be correct. Closure of these wounds earlier than the third day or later than the fifth day results in a higher failure rate of primary healing.

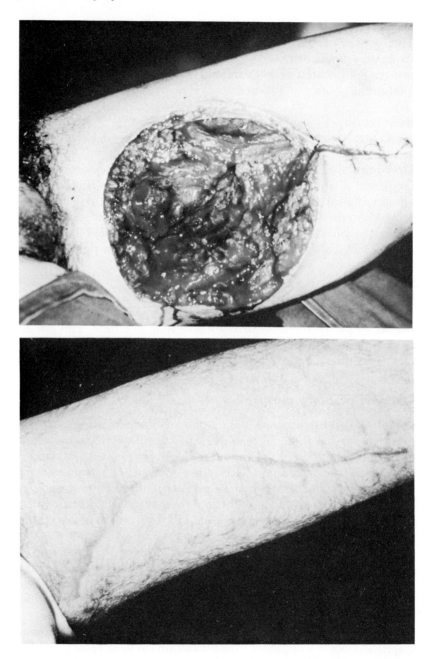

Fig. 5.1 a. Major missile wound of the thigh ready for delayed primary closure.
b. Thigh wound after delayed primary closure with primary healing. (Courtesy of
Professor G. W. Taylor)

At operation the wound is disturbed as little as possible, the edges are separated, any blood clot that is present is carefully removed and the wound may be gently irrigated with saline. Inevitably, these excised missile wounds tend to gape but this should not cause undue alarm provided there has been no significant loss of skin and subcutaneous tissues. The wound should be thoroughly inspected and any tiny tags of dead tissue which have been missed should be excised. It is imperative that haematoma formation should be avoided and therefore any bleeding points must be dealt with by hot packs or by using a small amount of fine non-absorbable suture material placed accurately on the bleeding point. In deeper wounds the track should be explored in case anything has been missed at the primary operation. No deep sutures are inserted and drainage is avoided where possible.

The skin edges may be undermined if necessary in order to provide cover without tension on the sutured edges. Such a procedure is safe in most areas up to 6–8 cm depth. Great care must be taken over haemostasis, the dead space must be obliterated as far as possible and the finished suture line should be lax and not under tension. Only fine suture material should be used for the skin. If there is any tension it means that there is a chance that the wound will break down. Therefore the wound should be closed as far as is possible without tension and the remaining area covered with split-skin graft. The sutured or grafted wound is then dressed and if it is on a limb it should be placed at rest in a padded plaster splint. It does not need to be disturbed for 10–14 days unless there is a definite indication. If there is any indication that all is not going well then the wound should be inspected in the theatre. Wounds which cannot be closed without tension must be covered with split thickness skin grafts. Open split thickness skin grafting is the method of choice for these missile wounds since good quality skin is readily available and the cosmetic result is preferable to that from mesh grafting.

Many wounds can only be closed satisfactorily by plastic methods and elaborate work of this nature is the responsibility of plastic surgeons.

We believe that 95 per cent of missile wounds are suitable for delayed closure and we would expect uncomplicated healing in over 90 per cent. (Fig 5.1)

The infected wound

This is usually due to inadequate primary wound excision. Such a wound will need a second operation to ensure that all dead tissue is excised. The appropriate antibiotic will have to be used and thorough drainage ensured. If it is only minor sepsis that responds rapidly to treatment, the wound may still be closed by delayed suture, but major sepsis will mean that the wound cannot be closed by delayed closure but will have to be closed by secondary suture or graft once the infection is completely under control.

When circumstances are poor there may be occasions when large numbers of untreated wounded may be admitted long after the infliction of the wound. When the time lag has been over 12 hours, major surgical interference is likely to do more harm than good and will spread sepsis and in such cases the basic minimum of surgery which involves the removal of dead tissues and the relief of tension, evacuation of haemato-mata and adequate drainage is advisable. This must be accomplished by incising the wound widely, removing all necrotic tissue and accessible foreign bodies. The appropriate antibiotic therapy is started.

The aim in surgery of missile wounds is to treat all such wounds prefer-ably within six hours and it is important to remember this time interval from wounding to surgery when planning surgical cover for a number of patients injured by missiles.

References and Further Reading

Cleveland, M. and Grove, J.A. (1945). Closure of wounds in compound fractures. *Journal of Bone and Joint Surgery*, **27** (3), 452–6.

Edlich, R.F. *et al.* (1969). Studies in the management of the contaminated wound. *American Journal of Surgery*, **117**, 323–9.

Fisher, D. (1953). Delayed primary closure of Korean war wounds. *Surgery, Gynecology and Obstetrics*, **96**, 696–703.

Lowry, K.F. and Curtis, G.M. (1950). Delayed suture in the management of wounds. *American Journal of Surgery*, **80**, 280–7.

Milligan, E.T.C. (1915). The early treatment of projectile wounds by excision of the damaged tissues. *British Medical Journal*, **1**, 1081.

Whelan, T.J., Burkhalter, W.E. and Gomez, A. (1968). Management of war wounds in *Advances in Surgery*, Vol. **3**, Year Book, Medical Publishers Inc., Chicago, pp. 227–349.

6

Vascular injuries

Injuries to major vessels require prompt surgical treatment if the tissues supplied by these vessels are to be salvaged. The diagnosis should be made early after wounding and preliminary treatment should be started immediately. Such patients carry a high priority for evacuation and ideally they should have an operation by a surgeon experienced in vascular techniques. The majority of acute vascular injuries that require surgical repair involve the peripheral vessels. Very few patients with injuries of major vessels of the abdominal or thoracic cavities ever survive to reach hospital but recent advances in rapid evacuation, particularly by helicopter, or where the injuries occur in an urban environment with good evacuation facilities have allowed some of these critically wounded patients to reach hospital alive. Delay will inevitably result in death as access cannot be gained to control the haemorrhage.

The major advances in vascular surgery that have been applied to bullet wounds have been made since the war in Korea. We now expect to have a significantly reduced rate of amputations of limbs following vascular trauma compared with the period of the early 1950s. Dramatic results following vascular repair can now be anticipated, but one must remember that reconstructive vascular surgery can only be performed effectively when proper surgical facilities and trained personnel are available. The operations are time-consuming and if there are multiple injuries, the patient's general condition must be evaluated as a whole and life must not be risked in order to save a limb. In addition, great judgement is necessary for weighing in the balance a limb which demonstrates injuries such that are severe enough to warrant immediate amputation rather than ligation or repair.

Military experience differs greatly from civilian experience in relation to the type of bullet creating wounds. The majority of civilian vascular injuries come from low velocity hand gun bullets or from shot gun injuries, whereas a large proportion of vascular injuries in war-time come from high velocity missiles. It is most important that the type of missile creating the vascular injury is known because as was shown in Chapter 2 the cavitational effects produced by high velocity missiles upon tissues creates damage to an artery even though the missile does not actually strike it. The mechanism consists of the artery taking part in the violent displacement of the cavitational process, causing essentially a severe stretch injury to the artery. This causes disruption of the intima, arterial wall dissection, intimal prolapse, obstruction of the lumen and thrombosis. If a high velocity bullet damages an artery directly, it does so by cutting it neatly but this is then followed by the gross displacement and violent distortion of the temporary cavity causing unseen damage to the ends of the artery.

The first aid treatment at the site of injury is to stop accessible haemorrhage. This may usually be effected sufficiently by pressure. If there is a large open wound with bleeding from the depths, this should be packed securely, ideally with an adequate sterile dressing, but if this is not available, with any piece of cloth, packing the material firmly into the depths of the wound and securing it in place with some form of bandage. Once bleeding has been stopped, the dressings should not be removed at a later stage until intravenous drips are in place, blood is available and running and the patient is in the Theatre. Experience has shown that once a dressing has been removed that had previously been effective it is extremely difficult to stop the bleeding on the second occasion.

Time is at a premium in vascular injuries. The vessels should be repaired and the vascular supply to the peripheral tissues restored as soon as possible. Ideally, all cases should be dealt with within 4–6 h and 10 h is the maximum time at which one might hope for a successful outcome. Attempts to restore the circulation after this time have little chance of success and, in addition, run the risks of the development of the 'crush syndrome' when the toxic metabolites of ischaemic tissue are released back into the circulation. Injuries to the blood vessel are of several types.

1. Lacerations
2. Transection
3. Avulsion
4. Contusions of the vessel wall with possible thrombosis or embolic occlusion
5. Expanding haematoma of the vessel wall
6. Extravascular compression or displacement from a haematoma or bony fragments

The differential diagnosis of vascular injury is sometimes difficult because a cold pulseless limb may result not only from direct arterial injury but from exposure, shock, spasm, crush injury and severe blows of the extremity. A wound which is in the vicinity of a large vessel should always arouse suspicion that the vessels may be injured. An accurate diagnosis may not be possible until after exploration, but the following signs and symptoms may be taken as presumptive evidence of arterial damage. The affected limb may be pale, mottled, waxy, cyanotic and cold. The pulse is usually absent, but the presence of a distal pulse does not definitely rule out arterial injury. Loss of voluntary motion of the limb, analgesia and muscle spasm may be present. External haemorrhage, which is obviously arterial, may or may not be present. The affected limb may be distinctly larger than the non-injured limb, particularly when a large haematoma is present.

Arterial spasm should not be diagnosed without exploration of the involved artery when there is a penetrating wound in its vicinity.

Technique of operation

The majority of arterial wounds from missiles are situated in the extremity and therefore the treatment of such a wound will be described. The limb is thoroughly prepared as for the excision of a soft tissue wound. In addition a potential donor site for the vein graft is prepared on the opposite limb. When the temporary dressing has been removed, direct pressure over the traumatized artery usually provides adequate temporary control of the haemorrhage. Adequate exposure of the injured vessel must always be ensured and the ends of the artery should be rapidly secured, first at the proximal end and then at the distal end of the damaged artery. Temporary occlusion of the artery can be maintained either with tapes or with non-crushing vascular clamps. The damaged tissues of the soft tissue wound are then thoroughly and rapidly excised. Excision of the damaged ends of the artery in a high velocity wound should be as conservative as possible. Only grossly injured artery should be removed and the vessel can be transected at a point where the wall appears grossly normal. Although there are microscopic changes in the arterial wall adjacent to the obviously damaged artery, extensive resection is not necessary and usually 0.5 cm of normal looking artery should be the maximum that has to be removed. The patency of the artery should be checked before repair is commenced by the passage of a Fogarty balloon catheter to clear any distal thrombus.

The procedure, thereafter, depends on whether the wound was created by a low or high velocity missile and whether the artery has been lacerated or transected. If the laceration of the artery has been caused by a low velocity missile, then repair by lateral suture or a vein patch may be performed. If the injury has been caused by a high velocity missile then even if there is just a laceration of the artery we must expect significant injury over a long segment of artery and the segment must be resected. Thrombus formation can occur on both sides of the arterial wound and its presence must be suspected. It is not usually possible to do an end-to-end anastomosis in any high velocity wound but it may be possible to do this by adequate mobilization of the ends of the artery when a low velocity missile has transected the vessel. Direct anastomosis should be performed, using synthetic vascular sutures 5-0 or 6-0 on fine, curved cutting needles. After placing stay sutures, a continuous suture is inserted through the full thickness of the vessel wall with sutures approximately 1 mm apart and 1 mm from each cut end of the artery. In small vessels of the size of the radial, ulnar or posterior tibial arteries, interrupted sutures should be used. A simple over and over continuous suture with accurate suturing joining intima to intima is satisfactory. Whilst the repair is being done, the lumen of the vessels should be repeatedly inspected to ensure that no fibrin, clots or fragments of intima are present. They should be removed by flushing the lumen with normal saline solution or citrate solution. The severed artery is usually in some degree of spasm and it is important that the continuous suture should not be too tight. Small leaks can usually be controlled by pressure alone but occasionally additional interrupted sutures may be necessary. With high velocity missiles the extent of the arterial damage is greater and after adequate wound excision the gap between the two arterial ends must be filled with a vein graft. Usually the saphenous vein is used for this and if the major venous return in the lower extremity is impaired, the saphenous vein graft should be obtained from the opposite leg. The vein grafts should be reversed to prevent obstruction of the blood flow by the valves and dilated by injection with saline under pressure; using the saphenous vein to make a panel graft is particularly useful for popliteal injuries. Synthetic prostheses should not be used for high velocity wounds because of the increased risk of infection. The presence of a large foreign body like a prosthesis causes disaster in many cases. Rarely a prosthesis may be utilized in large artery wounds of the thorax and abdomen caused by hand gun bullets but this is stressed as being a most unusual situation, when high velocity missiles are involved. The major vein that accompanies the damaged artery should be preserved whenever possible. Ligation is not desirable on theoretical and practical grounds and may result in disabling venous stasis of the extremity. Careful lateral repair, or indeed anastomosis of the vein, can be successfully performed and utilization of autologous vein graft in the venous sytem, particularly of the lower extremity, should also be considered because patency for even 24-72 h may give sufficient time to allow the establishment of futher collateral venous return.

After arterial repair, it is imperative that it be covered to prevent drying. An exposed artery repair will break down. It must, therefore, be covered by a flap of musculofascial tissue not only on the outer surface but also interposed between the arterial repair and a fracture.

Ligation is not a desirable method of treating arterial injuries and should be reserved for arterial damage in which repair is contraindicated because of the poor general condition of the patient and the inadvisability of the time spent in attempting a vascular repair. The expected incidence of gangrene of an extremity after ligation of the more critical arteries is predicted as follows: high axillary and high brachial ligation – 45–55 per cent, low brachial ligation –25 per cent, common femoral ligation – 80 per cent, superficial femoral ligation – 55 per cent, popliteal ligation – 75–100 per cent. Ligation of the profunda branches in the arm or the thigh in the absence of other arterial involvement in the same extremity does not run such a risk of acute arterial insufficiency.

Compound fractures are frequently associated with arterial injuries and may involve loss of bone length. Although unstable fractures can compromise the vascular repair, internal fixation of the fracture is contraindicated because of the increased risk of infection. External means of skeletal stabilization should be used, either skeletal traction or external bony fixation through bone proximal and distal to the site of the wound. When traction is used after an arterial repair, great care must be taken to ensure that there is no undue stressing at the site of the repair or compression by the fracture and careful readjustment should be ensured.

After arterial surgery, the injured limb should be kept neither elevated nor dependent but approximately at the level of the heart. Active muscle exercises are begun soon after operation whilst immobilization in bed is required, but as soon as other injuries permit, walking is allowed as soon as delayed primary closure of the soft tissue wounds has been completed.

Fasciotomies should be done at the time of arterial repair, particularly in relation to damage of the popliteal artery or vein or where there has been a delay between injury and repair. After operation careful watch must be maintained for the development of tightness in the fascial compartments or loss of sensation in the extremity. Fasciotomies should be performed at the first appearance of any swelling which compromises circulatory or neurological function.

Anticoagulation of the distal arterial tree is acceptable during the operation but systemic anticoagulation should be avoided during the operation and in the postoperative period. When it is available arteriography at the time of operation is helpful in order to rule out additional injuries or to indicate the presence and site of distal thrombus.

Overall, the amputation rate after ligation of major arteries following missile trauma was approximately 50 per cent. When routine arterial repair is done the amputation rate for missile injuries of arteries has fallen to about 13 per cent. The worst situation is still the popliteal artery where, even after arterial repair, the amputation rate is approximately 30 per cent.

References and Further Reading

Amato, J. J. *et al.* (1970). Vascular injuries, an experimental study of high and low velocity missile wounds. *Archives of Surgery*, **101**, 167–74.

DeBakey, M.E. and Simeone, F.A. (1946). Battle injuries of the arteries in World War II: analysis of 2471 cases. *Annals of Surgery*, **123**, 534–79.

Hughes, C.W. (1958). Arterial repair during the Korean War. *Annals of Surgery*, **147**, 555–61. ·

Livingstone, R.H. and Wilson, R.I. (1975). Surgery of violence VI. Gunshot wounds of the limbs. *British Medical Journal*, **1**, 667–9.

Makins, G.H. (1919). *Gunshot Injuries to the Blood Vessels*. John Wright and Sons, Bristol.

O'Reilly, M.J.G., Hood, J.M., Livingstone, R.H. and Irwin, J.W.S. (1978). Penetrating injuries of the popliteal artery. *British Journal of Surgery*, **65**, 789–92.

O'Reilly, M.J.G., Hood, J.M., Livingstone, R.H. and Irwin, J.W.S. (1979). Penetrating vascular injuries. *Journal of the Royal College of Surgeons of Edinburgh*, **24**, 213–20.

Rich, N.M. (1973). Vascular trauma. in Symposium of Trauma. *Surgical Clinics of North America* **53**, 1367–92.

Rich, N.M. and Hughes, C.W. (1972). The fate of prosthetic material used to repair vascular injuries in contaminated wounds. *Journal of Trauma*, **12**, 459–67.

Rich, N.M. and Spenser, F.C. (1978). *Vascular Trauma*. W.B. Saunders and Company, Philadelphia.

Rybeck, B., Lewis, D.H., Sandegard, J. and Seeman, T. (1975). The immediate circulatory response to high velocity missiles. *Journal of Trauma*, **15**, 328–35.

Schramek, A. and Hashmonai, M. (1977). Vascular injuries in the extremities in battle casualties. *British Journal of Surgery*, **64**, 644–8.

7
Amputations

There was a time when amputations formed the major part of war surgery and they still represent a small but important section of this type of work. We must remember the feat of Baron Larrey at the Battle of Borodino who performed two hundred amputations in twenty-four hours, and he was regarded as a conservative surgeon! In the preantiseptic period, gross suppuration was the rule and a compound fracture of a limb due to any form of trauma was regarded as an indication for prompt amputation. One is now much more optimistic but we must remember that optimism, in regard to conservative treatment can be carried too far.

The enormous number of amputations in World War I led to major advances in the techniques and development of prostheses. For example, in this country the study of over 40 000 amputees under the authority of the Ministry of Pensions provided evidence from which surgeons of the day were able to mould their current practice.

Amputations were described by Gillis as essentially a means of repairing the remains of a limb and of making what is left as useful as possible as soon as possible. It may be forced upon the surgeon by the severity of the injury or its complications, or it may be chosen in preference to a limb that is, or will become a serious handicap to the patient concerned.

During World War II the Army Medical Directorate issued instructions which emphasized the need for the conservation of all tissues when dealing with severely injured casualties in the front line and casualty clearing stations. Definitive surgery was discouraged until the patient had reached advance base hospitals with the exception of those cases who had to be dealt with by the Field Surgical Units. When performing amputations in the battle zone, it is justifiable to sacrifice only that amount of the limb necessary to save life and to combat infection. Surgeons in the field should not concern themselves too much as to whether to amputate at the optimum site, they must be content with amputating at the lowest possible level. They should constantly keep in mind the saving of life as well as of limb. The following principles must be emphasized.

1. Emergency operations should be performed through or immediately above the level of the trauma without regard for the ultimate prosthesis.
2. The site should depend more upon the level of bone injury than on the highest level of the soft tissue loss.
3. Viable skin must never be sacrificed; the preservation of skin beyond the level of amputation permits early healing, combats infection and improves the definitive surgery if it becomes necessary. Many war time amputees have not had to have reamputations and many of these cases are wearing comfortable artificial limbs to date.
4. The amputation must always be as simple as possible.

The object of the operation is to prevent infection of the soft tissue wound and thus prevent infection of the bony fragments. This is accomplished by the two-stage operation on soft tissue wounds already described, i.e. the primary operation is wound excision, the secondary operation is delayed primary closure. The time of the initial operation should be as early as possible after wounding and every effort should be made to do it within six hours. The hazards of primary suture in dirty trauma cases must be constantly remembered; the risk of infection, particularly gas gangrene, with subsequent morbidity and mortality makes this method unacceptable.

The surgeon must aim to provide a soundly healed comfortable stump as soon as possible. With a fresh injury it may be practicable to carry out a formal amputation at one of the sites of election, that is the site preferred by the limb-fitting surgeon, but we must remember that it is usually possible to fit a useful appliance to any well-healed stump. When there is infection, and this means any dirty wound such as result from most kinds of trauma, flaps may be cut during amputation but must be left open for delayed primary closure.

All amputations should be done through uninfected and uninjured tissues but there is no need to go high above the level of infection. Experience in war-time has shown that bone infection quickly disappears with adequate drainage, and all amputations afford excellent drainage. If the wounds are left open after the flaps have been cut, infection settles down and the case may well not require secondary amputation. The level of bone injury or any infection should determine the level of amputation, not the level of the wound. At the end of World War II, because of the success in obtaining delayed primary skin closure, it was realized that as much bone as possible should be retained. Previously it had been thought that bone fragments without attachments were liable to infection. This is certainly true if the wound is allowed to heal by granulation, but by obtaining healing with delayed primary closure aided by antibiotics, wound infection has been largely overcome. Meticulous cleaning of bone fragments in the wound using a curette and copious irrigation with saline is essential at the time of wound excision. Large bony fragments without attachments must also be retained for the simple reason that if they are removed a gap results and this complicates the later treatment and usually results in shortening of the limb.

Amputation as a result of bullet and fragment wounds and from explosive blast can usually be divided into three types: traumatic amputation; early surgical amputation and late surgical amputation.

Traumatic amputation

This is defined as an amputation occuring at the moment of injury. The term is also used for a virtual amputation when the limb is only attached by a little skin and soft tissue. The mass movement of air resulting from explosive blast is the most important cause of traumatic amputation. This blast wave can result from conventional explosive devices like bombs, mines, shells, grenades and from home-made bombs. When explosions take place in confined surroundings particularly if the compartments are rigid, then the incidence of traumatic amputation resulting from the incident may well exceed 30 per cent. This poses enormous problems for the rescue services dealing with the extraction, triage, treatment and evacuation of the wounded.

In cases of traumatic amputation when the wound is clean and seen within six hours, formal amputation higher up may be considered, skin flaps may be cut but should be left open. If the wound is dirty or seen after six hours delay, then the dirty and necrotic tissues should be excised and protruding bone trimmed, all viable tissue should be preserved, particularly skin. The wounds should then be closed by delayed primary closure 4–5 days later.

Early surgical amputation

High velocity bullets and explosive blast injuries may cause such severe damage that immediate amputation becomes inevitable. It is usually required when the degree of destruction is so gross that there is no alternative. The limb may be so mangled, with extensive comminuted fractures, neurovascular damage and gross lacerations that there is no room for doubt and an amputation should be performed immediately. If the limb has been trapped and crushed for a long period of time, particularly over 4–6 h, and the leg is cold and pallid with solid oedema present, than the toxic effect of the absorption of damaged muscle products will almost certainly produce the 'crush syndrome'. Under these circumstances, primary amputation as a life-saving operation may become necessary. Burns of the limb that destroy the whole skin may be an indication for early surgical amputation but no burn injury is to be considered hopeless unless the main vascular supply to the lower limb is completely destroyed.

A toilet amputation alone may be required but usually it is a far bigger procedure and the wounds must be treated according to the surgical principles already described. All dead tissue must be thoroughly excised, dead bone must be removed but as much viable bone as possible should be preserved in the first instance providing that it appears practicable to cover it with some form of skin at a later stage. The amputation should be performed through or immediately above the level of bone injury and viable skin must never be sacrificed. The healthy, but contaminated, tissues must then be left open and covered with a bulky, fluffed up dressing which will absorb all the fluid discharges from the wound. Primary suture must not be performed. If the skin looks as though it will retract then one suture over the bulky dressing should be enough to hold the ends in a reasonable position. The wound should be inspected 4–5 days later and delayed primary closure should be possible in most cases using a combination of suture and split-skin graft. If the stump proves unsatisfactory later on in terms of its shape, length or the quality of skin cover, then a definitive operation can be performed at a later date. Thin unstable scars that may result from split skin grafting under these circumstances can readily be replaced by plastic surgery procedures such as a cross leg flap or tube pedicle.

In the upper limb the preservation of all possible length is most important and in particular any skin with intact sensation should be retained. In the lower limb any length of stump below the knee joint is worth preserving, at least in the first instance. When the wounds are relatively clean and have been seen within six hours of injury, formal amputation at the site of election may be done but one must always remember the risk that is attached and even under these circumstances it is most important not to perform primary suture.

Late surgical amputation

Surgical judgement and assessment of the patient are particularly important when it has been decided to try and preserve a badly injured limb. A preservative operation may have made great demands on the surgeon's skill and understandably this may create in him, and the patient, the sense of obligation to tackle any setbacks that might occur. Sloughs, sequestra, haemorrhage, infection and skin problems come to be regarded as challenges to be conquered. When faced with a limb for which salvage is no more than a possibility it is only fair to make this quite clear to the patient and to stress that primary salvage must be regarded as purely provisional and that apparently minor complications that occur may well seal the fate of the limb. Prepared in this way from the beginning, many patients accept late surgical amputation with resignation and, not being sustained by false hope, apply themselves without delay to learning their new way of life. It is at times like this that experience is so important and second opinions so helpful but a plea must be made for taking a decision to amputate within a reasonable space of time; nothing is more disappointing for the patient than many months of wasted time when the chances of success were so slim in the first place. The indications for late surgical amputation may be grouped under a number of headings.

Orthopaedic
Even when the most energetic efforts have been made, non-union may still occur and lead to late amputation.

Vascular
This is probably the commonest complication and one which is apparent quite soon after any operation to repair the blood vessels. Recent advances in vascular surgery have resulted in a significant reduction in the rate of amputation of limbs as a result of trauma. Vascular injuries require prompt surgical intervention, the aim being to repair the vessel and restore arterial flow to the affected part at the earliest possible moment. A repair that has been done and which fails is usually made apparent to both patient and surgeon in quite a short space of time and there is little problem over the decision for late amputation.

Nerve
When nerves have been repaired as a secondary procedure after primary healing of the wound has taken place, there is an inevitable delay until time has elapsed to allow regeneration of the nerve. When nerve repair does not give useful function, amputation may still be required. This will be a much later event and will be a formal amputation done with the full co-operation of the prosthetist and the Limb Fitting Centre

Sepsis
This is particularly important where gas gangrene is concerned. In spite of wound excision, antibiotics and hyperbaric oxygen therapy the disease may not be controlled and amputation is a life-saving measure. The perils of preserving such a damaged limb which is an irretrievable culture medium for toxin-producing bacteria must be considered most carefully. Evidence of renal impairment may be an indication for the excision

of necrotic tissue or, indeed, for the early amputation of a necrotic limb.

Rehabilitation following amputation as a result of bullet wounds or blast injury requires the development of maximum mobility and use of the prosthesis which will be provided by the Limb Fitting Centres. Overall progress is fostered in special units where the competitive spirit is encouraged. Progress and success after the severe physical and psychological trauma of amputation depends above all on morale. To achieve this the close co-operation is required between all who are concerned with limb amputation and limb replacement.

Part 3
Regional Management

8
Limbs

We must expect somewhere between 60 and 75 per cent of all missile wounds and blast injuries to involve the upper or lower extremities. Such wounds form the bulk of those to be treated and are, therfore, usually the first type of missile wound that a surgeon is likely to be called upon to treat (Fig 8.1). Using surgical methods and techniques that have stood the test of time we expect to get good results from extremity wounds and the mortality is low. The management of a compound fracture is very similar to that of a soft tissue wound already described but with the special addition of the injury to bone and any associated injuries to blood vessels and nerves.

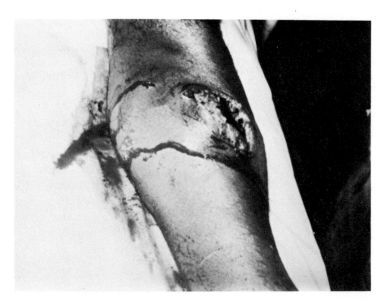

Fig. 8.1 a. Penetrating wound of the leg from high velocity fragments from a mortar bomb.

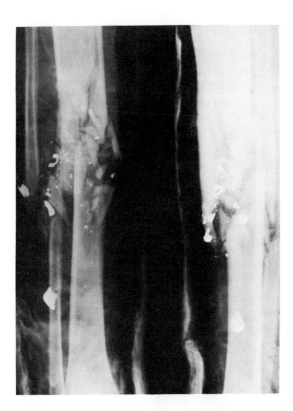

Fig. 8.1 b. X-ray showing comminuted fracture of the tibia and fibula.

First-aid

Any open missile wounds should be covered by a sterile or clean dressing before the application of splints. Splintage should be simple, effective and designed to immobilize the limb in order to reduce pain and to prevent further damage to the soft tissues by the fractured bone. In the upper extremity, the arm may be bandaged to the side or a sling may be used. In the lower extremity, the leg can usually be splinted, after padding the bony points, to the good leg or it may be splinted using some sort of emergency splint either rigid or of the inflatable type. Particular attention should be paid to examination of the blood and nerve supply to the limb before the application of splints.

Management in the casualty or emergency department

There may well be other associated injuries and the sum total of these must be evaluated and the general condition of the patient assessed. Resuscitation measures must be taken immediately, the wounds examined and an assessment made of the vascular and neurological state of the extremity distal to the injury. Tetanus toxoid and penicillin should be given and an intravenous drip set up if necessary. Radiographs are usually possible at this stage and give a good idea of the extent of the injury and the likely type of missile. It is most important to try and find out whether the missile was likely to be of high velocity type. Quite commonly a small entry and exit wound in a limb will look the same whether it comes from a low velocity pistol bullet or a high velocity rifle bullet and yet there is a world of difference between the damage caused within the limb by these two different types of missile (Fig 8.2 and 8.3).

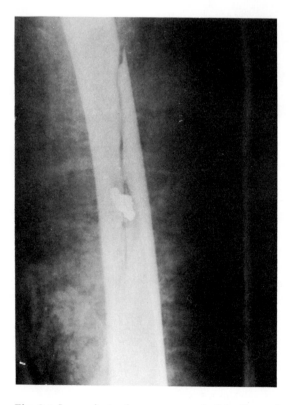

Fig. 8.2 Low velocity fragment wound of the femur showing a simple crack in the bone.

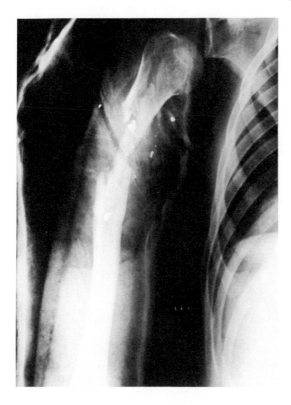

Fig. 8.3 High velocity fragment wound of the upper humerus.

Management at operation

It is permissible to put a tourniquet into place and this may be used in the earliest phase of the operation until complete control of major bleeding has been obtained. It must then be released to confirm viability of damaged soft tissues. The approach should be through generous skin incisions usually in the long axis of the extremity with deviation in the usual manner if the incision crosses a flexion crease. Deep fascia must then be divided throughout the length of the incision to allow the wound to be opened widely. There is usually a large haematoma with a lot of pulped muscle tissue, debris and foreign material. Bone will commonly be shattered into a number of pieces, most of these have either soft tissue attachment or periostium. Tiny fragments of bone without any attachment should be discarded. All other fragments should be cleaned thoroughly using a curette and copious irrigation and replaced (Fig. 8.4). Any large detached fragment, particularly those that contribute to maintaining the length of the bone, should be cleaned and replaced. The major

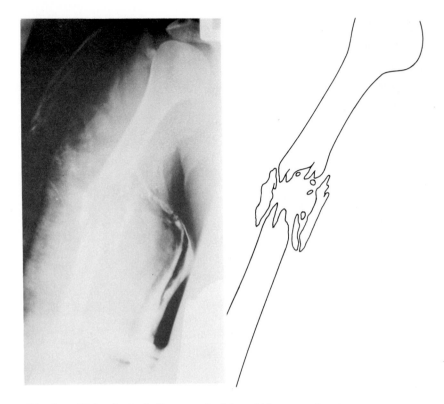

Fig. 8.4a High velocity bullet wound of the mid-humerus showing gross destruction of bone and tiny fragments at the periphery of the temporary cavity.

bone ends should be brought roughly into line, and the soft tissues are excised in the fashion already described. Repairs of the major blood vessel to the limb must be performed at the earliest stages of the operation when they are indicated. Any nerves that are severed are marked and their position noted; no attempt is made at primary repair. The same treatment is necessary for severed tendons, but any damaged parts should be excised and loose or frayed edges trimmed. Internal fixation of bone is not advisable in these injuries, even when required to protect an accompanying arterial anastomosis. However, external fixation using pins placed through normal tissues above and below the fractures is permitted and recommended (Fig. 8.5).

Decompression of the four osseofascial compartments of the leg is of particular importance following the severe trauma of penetrating high velocity missile wounds. Through each of these four compartments of the leg runs a neurovascular bundle which may be damaged by an excessive rise in pressure causing a compartment syndrome with resultant

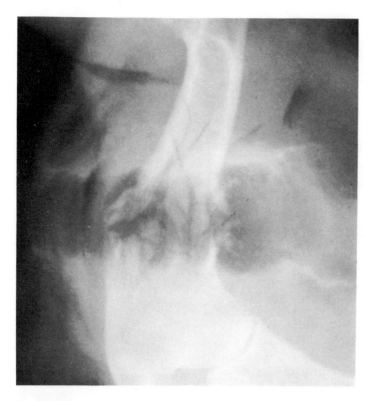

Fig. 8.4b High-speed radiograph of the cavitation resulting from a rifle bullet hitting bone. Note the gross displacement of the many small fragments which are later pulled back roughly into place by the elasticity of the surrounding tissues and their periosteal attachments. (Crown Copyright Reserved)

ischaemic contracture. Knowledge of the anatomy of each compartment is important in avoiding damage to the neurovascular bundles during fasciotomy. At the time of excision of the wound, it is usually possible to deal with decompression of two compartments and a further incision will be required to deal with the remaining two compartments. The four compartments involved are the anterior, lateral, superficial posterior and deep posterior. Decompression of all four compartments can be performed through a standard two incision fasciotomy. It can also be performed by fibulectomy through a single incision. The double incision method is perfectly adequate and is simple to perform.

The anterior and lateral compartments are approached through a single longitudinal incision 15 cm in length placed halfway down the leg 2 cm anterior to the shaft of the fibula. This places the incision approximately over the anterior intermuscular septum dividing the

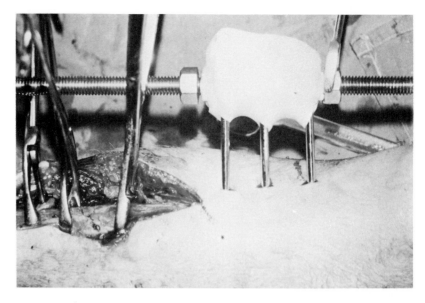

Fig. 8.5 a. Immobilization of the fracture caused by a missile wound using an external fixation device.

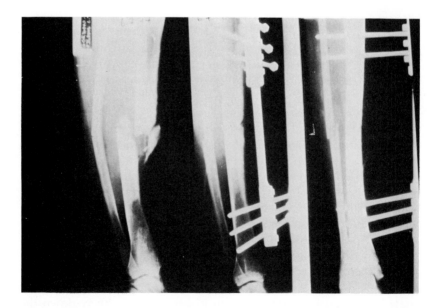

Fig. 8.5 b. X-ray showing the Denham external fixator in position. (Courtesy of Mr Robin Denham)

anterior and lateral compartments and allows easy access to both. The septum is identified, a nick is made in the fascia of the anterior compartment mid-way between the septum and the crest of the tibia. The fascia is opened proximally and distally with long blunt pointed scissors. The lateral compartment fasciotomy is made in line with the shaft of the fibula.

The two posterior compartments are best approached through a single longitudinal incision 15 cm in length in the distal part of the leg placed 2 cm posterior to the palpable posteromedial edge of the tibia. The deep posterior compartment is readily accessible and its fascia is opened distally and proximally under the belly of the soleus muscle. Through the same incision the fascia of the superficial posterior compartment is opened along a line 2 cm posterior and parallel to the incision of the deep compartment. The wounds are left open for delayed closure.

At the end of the operation, having checked that all dead tissue has been excised and that there is adequate decompression of the compartments enclosed by the deep fascia, the wound must be left open. Gauze should be placed across these wounds and this should be covered with a bulky, fluffed up gauze dressing in order to allow completely free drainage. Fixation of the dressing should not be done with any form of circumferential strapping; plaster slabs may then be applied. If a formal padded plaster is applied it must be very well padded and must be split down to the skin prior to leaving the theatre.

If there is a definite indication the wound must be inspected, otherwise it should be left alone for five days after the initial surgery. At this inspection the wound should be clean and healthy. There may be a small amount of dead tissue which should be removed but this is a reflection on the inadequacy of the first operation. At this time the oedema of the tissues around the wound should be settled and it is the optimum time for delayed primary closure. In wounds of the lower leg, however, it may be more advisable to leave the wound for nearer ten days before attempting delayed primary closure. At operation the wound is closed by suture if this is possible without creating too much tension in the skin, otherwise it may be closed in part by skin graft (Fig. 8.6). One must always remember that in these wounds the prime consideration must be the healing of the soft tissues first before tackling any problem to do with the bone and the nerves (Fig. 8.7).

The immobilization of the fracture by plaster techniques, by external bone fixation devices or by skeletal traction will continue along conventional lines.

It is vital that constant vigilance is kept at all stages of treatment following missile wounds of the limbs in order to detect the onset of vascular complications or infection. A rise in tissue tension caused by the effects of trauma to the tissues may be followed by an ischaemic necrosis of muscle and this can occur even in the presence of a distal pulse. In addition to external constricting factors such as the effects of hard, dried blood on the dressings or circumferential strapping, inadequate decompression of the deep fascia, in particular at primary wound excision, may result in such increased tissue tension. The common sites for closed compartment compressions are in the forearm and in the anterior tibial compartment of the leg. Severe and increasing pain beneath plasters, in association with pain on passive extension of the fingers or passive plantar

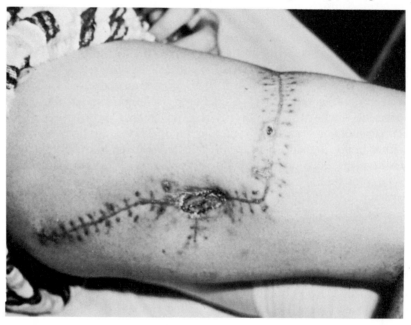

Fig. 8.6 High velocity wound of the thigh 10 days after delayed primary closure by suture and by skin graft.

flexion of the toes, is an indication of this tension and imminent muscle necrosis. Remember this is particularly true of the missile wounds of the fibula for this bone is connected to all three fascial compartments of the lower leg and it may be necessary to decompress all of them by division of the deep fascia in order that an increase in tension will not return. In a similar way great care has to be taken over the injuries of the forearm. Increasing pain beneath a plaster may also indicate the presence of infection. The presence of pain that is out of proportion to the injury, especially if it is associated with a rising pulse rate demands immediate inspection of the limb in the theatre with complete removal of all plaster and dressings in order to exclude the possibility of gas gangrene.

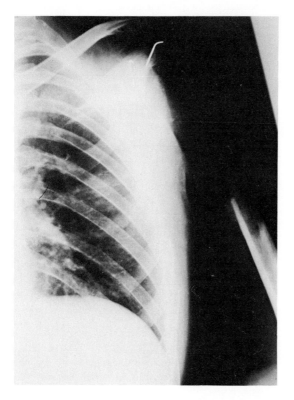

Fig. 8.7. This man lost the whole shoulder joint, part of the scapula, and the upper end of the humerus when he was struck by an accidental discharge from a Carl Gustav antitank practice missile. The remains of the arm have good vascular and nerve function and the main problem is that of reconstruction and to maintain length of the upper limb. (Courtesy of Colonel J. Coull).

Joint injuries

The principles of the actual surgery of a penetrating wound of the joint are the same as those previously described for wounds of soft tissues and bone, but particular care must be taken to apply extra precautions in order to try and prevent any significant infection which is so disastrous for joint function (Fig. 8.8). The wound of a joint may be extended as necessary, or a separate standard arthrotomy incision may be required. Here again a tourniquet may be placed on the limb for the early stages of the operation. All loose bony fragments, detached or badly damaged cartilage, foreign bodies, debris and blood clots should be removed. The damaged tissues must be excised. All recesses of the joint must be thoroughly explored to make sure that no damaged tissue or foreign body is left behind. Then the joint is irrigated thoroughly with saline until

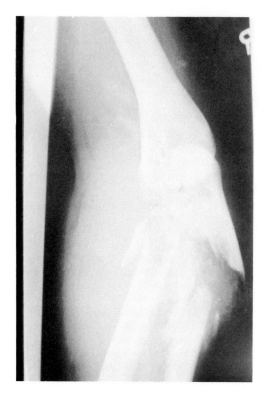

Fig. 8.8 High velocity bullet wound of the elbow showing the gross disruption of the joint and a comminuted fracture of the radius and ulna.

all remaining minor debris has been flushed out. The synovium should be closed and the remaining tissues left open for delayed primary closure. If the synovium cannot be closed, then the capsule should be closed, and if the capsule cannot be closed, the chances are the joint has been so damaged that little function is likely. Joint injuries should be dressed in the usual fashion after leaving the superficial tissues completely open and the joint immobilized in the position of function using a well padded plaster that is split down to the skin. It is particularly important to remove any metallic debris from the missile, especially lead, that may have been impacted in part of the joint's surface. This is because if lead is left behind it will leach out into the synovial fluid and cause a lead arthritis. After delayed primary closure and a period of immobilization, the joint can be mobilized cautiously. If, in spite of adequate treatment, infection ensues then the appropriate antibiotic may be administered systematically and by continuous intra-articular catheter perfusion. If a joint wound is seen after a considerable delay and infection has already occurred, emergency treatment is still indicated with excision of all devitalized tissues including those within the joint, the removal of all foreign bodies, debris and the release of pus. This should be followed by copious irrigation, systemic antibiotics and intra-articular catheter perfusion of antibiotics. Occasionally the function of such a joint may be saved.

References and Further Reading

Cleveland, M., Manning, J. G. and Stewart, W. J. (1951). Care of battle casualties and injuries involving bones and joints. *Journal of Bone and Joint Surgery* **33A,** 517–27.

Furlong, R. and Clark, J. M. P. (1947). Missile wounds involving bone. *British Journal of Surgery*. War Surgery Supplement **2,** 291–310.

Guthrie, G. T. (1815) *On Gunshot Wounds of the Extremities*. Longman, London.

Hampton, O. P. (1951). *Wounds of the Extremities in Military Surgery*. Henry Kimpton, London.

Howland, W. S. and Ritchey, J. S. (1971). Gunshot fractures in civilian practice. *Journal of Bone and Joint Surgery* **53A,** 47-55.

Livingstone, R. H. and Wilson, R. I. (1975). Gunshot wounds of the limbs. *British Medical Journal* **1,** 667-9.

9
Abdomen and pelvis

Abdominal wounds require urgent treatment. The patient who has been wounded in the abdomen is almost certain to die unless he is operated upon. Speed is essential, for the outlook is grave unless he is operated upon early and mortality increases with increasing time that has elapsed from injury to operation. A high index of suspicion must be maintained, because those wounded in the trunk, thighs or buttocks may well have a wound that penetrates the abdominal cavity.

The severity and the prognosis of abdominal wounds varies with the causal agents and on the viscera that are damaged. Bullets from hand guns are usually of low velocity, they have a tendency to cause small entrance wounds and to be retained within the body, they usually cause simple damage to viscera by virtue of their penetration but without extensive tissue disruption. On the other hand, rifle bullets have a high velocity and may well pass right through the body causing a perforating wound. If, however, the rifle bullet is unstable or fragments easily, it tends to be retained within the tissues and therefore gives up much more energy than a comparable stable bullet which passes straight through. There is always a tendency for rifle bullets to cause severe disruptive wounds with widespread damage at a considerable distance from the actual track of the missile.

Fragments from any form of explosive device, whether it be conventional shell, bomb or rocket or a home-made bomb, may be large or small but they are usually multiple and they have a high initial velocity which rapidly falls off due to their irregular, unstreamlined shapes. The entry wounds are usually ragged and the damage that they do to the tissues depends upon their velocity. High velocity fragments cause damage similar to high velocity bullets and low velocity fragments cause damage similar to low velocity bullets. Very tiny fragments from explosive devices, which are travelling at high-velocity, may produce minute superficial wounds which can be associated with suprisingly severe internal damage. Intra-abdominal injury can easily be overlooked from such tiny wounds unless the examination is most careful and observation is maintained in all suspected cases.

The blast pressure wave may damage viscera by direct or indirect trauma. Pure blast effects to the abdomen are unusual in explosions in air except very close to the centre of the explosion. However, under-water explosions tend to cause closed abdominal injury at considerable distances. In addition to petechial haemorrhages throughout the affected tissues, there may be multiple ruptures of various hollow viscera. The caecum, large intestine, small intestine, bladder and stomach may be in-jured in that order of frequency. The blast wave may throw the victim violently to the ground or he may be crushed by falling debris and these effects may also cause intra-abdominal injury, especially to the fixed organs such as the liver, spleen, pancreas and the bowel at its points of fixation.

The treatment of penetrating missile injuries of the abdomen is surgical and the most important aspect of management, at the site of injury, is to evacuate the patient rapidly to hospital. In these patients shock is com-pounded of many elements, the most serious of which, bleeding from lacerated mesenteric vessels and solid organs and leakage from damaged viscera into the peritoneal cavity, cannot be combated by ordinary methods of resuscitation and early operation is required as part of the resuscitation process.

First-aid in missile wounds of the abdomen involves the application of a clean dressing to the wound, in particular to any viscera that may be protruding, and rapid evacuation. If there is going to be any delay in evacuation and facilities are available, an intravenous drip using Hart-mann's solution should be commenced after taking blood for grouping and cross-matching.

When the patient reaches the casualty or emergency department of the hospital, he is assessed according to the urgency with which he requires resuscitation and surgery and if a number of patients arrive together they must be allocated a priority for treatment. In abdominal wounds the com-monest cause of death is from haemorrhage. Patients wounded in the abdomen who are shocked and are resuscitated by electrolyte solution, plasma or blood tend to relapse within three or four hours. A second transfusion does not resuscitate them as well as the first and, indeed, may fail to render them fit for anything but a hurried operation. Major haemorrhage demands treatment at the earliest possible moment, whereas the closure of intestinal leaks is a less urgent matter. Antibiotic therapy must start immediately with intravenous benzyl penicillin and ampicillin together with intravenous metronidazole.

Penetration of the abdominal cavity is usually readily diagnosed when bullets or other missiles are involved. Apart from evidence of visceral damage, the welling up of blood, intestinal contents or urine or pro-trusion of omentum from a wound is sufficient proof that the abdominal cavity has been penetrated. In perforating wounds the direction of the track will give an indication of viscera likely to have been injured, whereas in single penetrating wounds an estimate of the direction of the track is difficult without knowledge of where a foreign body lies. Radiographic screening or anterior-posterior and lateral films give the needed information to determine the track of the missile. The importance of wounds in the buttocks or upper thighs cannot be over-stressed for these are often accompanied by injury to the rectum, bladder, peritoneum and pelvic vessels.

Operation

The best time for operation, on a penetrating abdominal injury, is the earliest at which the patient can stand it. Cases where haemorrhage is the chief problem should take precedence over those in which intestinal perforation dominates the picture. The wounds in the abdominal wall, like all other wounds, should be excised but time must not be wasted on this step when the clinical picture suggests that major intra-abdominal bleeding has occurred; such wound excision can be carried out on completion of the intraperitoneal operation. Usually a full laparotomy incision should be made. For severe injuries a generous full length midline incision is quickest and best. The right or left paramedian, or rectus-splitting incision, are all good. The oblique or transverse incision in the lateral aspect of the abdomen are acceptable but transverse incisions across the rectus muscle are bad in high velocity missile wounds and are often followed by ventral herniae.

After the patient is anaesthetized a catheter is passed into the bladder to see if there is any blood in the urine.

The abdominal cavity usually contains free fluid, blood or intestinal contents which must be rapidly evacuated before the damage can be traced. Haemorrhage is the chief cause of death and must be dealt with first. Peritonitis is the secondary and the less urgent danger. When the abdomen is full of blood, the most likely sources of the bleeding are the mesentery of the small intestine, the liver, spleen, kidney and pancreas, and the large veins of the posterior abdominal wall. The bleeding points must be found and ligated with fine thread or Dexon; catgut ligatures are prone to slip and catgut knots readily come undone when the parts are subsequently handled and this leads to further blood loss, subperitoneal or mesenteric haematomata that obscure the parts to be repaired. Injuries of the large blood vessels are usually lethal, but occasionally such a severely injured patient may get to hospital in time to be saved. Severe bleeding from the liver can be controlled temporarily by Pringle's manoeuvre but as a rule haemorrhage from tears in the liver has ceased by the time the abdomen is opened or can be arrested temporarily by light packing. If necessary, the search may be made easier by delivering the intestines on to the abdominal wall into a plastic bag. When haemorrhage has been dealt with, the surgeon must find and repair all perforations in the alimentary tract. All perforations must be found and to do this it is necessary to have a logical approach to examination of the gut. The viscera in the line of the missile track should be examined first but all organs that may have been injured must be inspected thoroughly. It is usual to postpone any repair until all the injuries have been discovered and assessed together since resection may, on occasions, be more sensible than multiple individual repairs.

The small intestine is the part most frequently injured and will usually be examined first and repaired before dealing with the colon. Loops many feet apart in continuity may well lie adjacent to each other in the abdomen so that the whole length of the small bowel should be inspected methodically from caecum to duodenojejunal junction. Each perforation or tear is marked with forceps applied to its edges and then each perforation is repaired. When the mesentry has been torn from the bowel or there are multiple perforations in a short length, resection should be considered.

After the small intestine, the stomach, colon and solid viscera should be examined each in turn. A retroperitoneal haemorrhage, in the region of the ascending or descending colon or signs of the wound track being in the vicinity, should lead to a most careful search for any perforation of the bare areas of the colon. It may be necessary to mobilize the colon by incising the parietal peritoneum lateral to the ascending and descending colon and stripping medially in order to expose the posterior surface.

When examining the stomach, the posterior wall must be exposed by opening the gastrocolic omentum. The duodenum can be inspected after the stomach and this, like the colon, has a bare area that may have been injured. The duodenum may be mobilized by Kocher's manoeuvre in order to examine it more closely.

Finally, the pelvis should be examined for injury to the rectum or bladder and where the lesion in the latter is large enough to admit the finger, its cavity should be explored for any foreign body, at the same time damage to the base of the bladder can be assessed and dealt with.

When all the lesions have been found and considered together they must be repaired individually by methods that will be considered in greater detail later. At the end of the operation the abdominal cavities should be mopped clean, the abdominal incision should be closed in layers and this should be reinforced by tension sutures of stainless steel or synthetic materials inserted as the first step in the closure and tied as the last over short lengths of rubber tubing. If there is a grossly contaminated wound the cutaneous portion of the abdominal incision should be left open with a sterile dressing in place and it should be closed by delayed primary closure.

Large abdominal wounds resulting from high velocity missiles should be thoroughly excised and if the resultant defect cannot be closed without tension by local soft tissues, then synthetic mesh may have to be used for closure even in the presence of contamination.

After all operations for the repair of penetrating abdominal wounds the abdominal cavity must be thoroughly drained. The drains should be led down to areas of soiling, damage or extensive repair. The drains may be of plastic material or rubber; they may be tubes or corrugated but whatever type they are, they should be brought out through separate, generous incisions rather than through the original wound or the laparotomy wound and should be so placed that gravity drainage is facilitated. Good pelvic drainage should be achieved by excising the tip of the coccyx, placing drains between sacrum and rectum. The retroperitoneal tissues are very vulnerable because cellulitus and clostridial invasion from contaminated contents are likely. Whenever the ascending or descending colon has been injured, the retroperitoneal space should be generously drained, any blood clot and debris being thoroughly cleaned out first. Drainage is best achieved through separate incisions posteriorly in the flanks, and the drainage tubes can be passed upwards and towards the kidney regions with separated tubes running medially.

Regional injuries

Stomach

The stomach is wounded in about 10–15 per cent of all penetrating abdominal wounds. They may be small or large perforations, linear tears or complete transections. Wounds of the stomach carry a high mortality because they are commonly associated with injuries to neighbouring organs such as the transverse colon, jejunum, liver, spleen, pancreas and kidney but isolated wounds are relatively benign. Wounds of the body should be excised and closed with a double layer of sutures; any repair which leaves a narrowed lumen near the pylorus may require the addition of a gastrojejunostomy.

Duodenum

Wounds of the duodenum are not frequently encountered by the surgeon because of the high associated mortality. Injury to the duodenum is seldom isolated because it is almost always associated with significant injuries of pancreas, liver, stomach, kidney and great vessels; such patients commonly have severe and life-threatening haemorrhage. Minor wounds of the duodenum should be treated by excision and then closed transversely after thorough mobilization of the duodenum and examination of the posterior wall. More severe wounds may be treated by partial resection and gastrojejunostomy. Particular attention must be paid to keeping the duodenum decompressed after operation and to the drainage at the site of the anastomosis and the retroduodenal area.

Small intestine

The small intestine is wounded in about 30 per cent of abdominal cases and almost always the wounds are multiple. The perforations are commonly sealed by pouting mucous membrane so that they may not leak very much. Blood in the peritoneum is far more characteristic of small intestine injury than is presence of intestinal contents. Perforations of the small intestine should be closed by suture, the edges need only a small amount of trimming and a single layer of interrupted invaginating sutures is usually enough. Resection of small gut should be performed when a group of perforations is so close that their repair would overlap, when so many injuries are found in a given segment that resection of the loop will save time and when the injury is on the mesenteric border. It may also be necessary when the viability of a loop of gut has been impaired by crushing, by thrombosis of the vessels or by detachment of its mesentery. End-to-end anastomosis should be done by the method which the surgeon normally practises (Fig. 9.1 and 9.2).

Colon

Wounds of the colon occur almost as frequently as those of the small intestine. They are usually more serious because the blood supply is not so good, the contents of the large bowel escape more readily and are highly infective; there are often retroperitoneal injuries which are easily overlooked and cellulitis, which is often an anaeorobic infection, is a common and fatal complication. Perforations in the colon should be looked for carefully as those that are in the fixed portion and on the mesenteric aspect of the transverse colon are difficult to demonstrate and are easily missed. Thorough exploration requires incision of the lateral peritoneal reflection in order to mobilize the colon and permit direct inspection of the retroperitoneal areas. The absence of peritoneal soiling does not preclude perforations of the colon. Any part of the wall of the colon which is contused or discoloured should be repaired, resected or exteriorized. A haematoma in the mesocolen or in the right or left paracolic gutters calls for a minute examination of the adjacent bowel

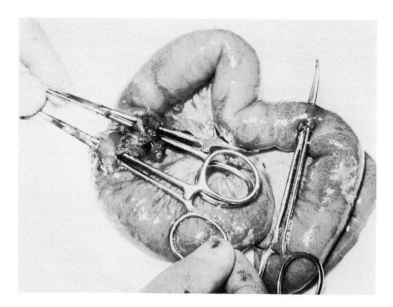

Fig. 9.1 Multiple penetrating wounds of the small intestine.

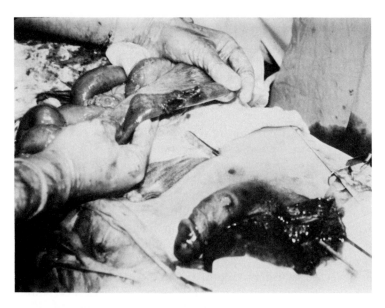

Fig. 9.2 Wounds of the small bowel may be only part of a very complicated process of wounding. In this patient fragments from a mine caused traumatic amputation of a foot, penetrated the perineum, the bladder, small bowel, large bowel, liver and finally ended in the lung.

wall. A faeculant smell may draw attention to a hole that can scarcely be seen. The treatment of colon injuries is based on the known insecurity of suture and the dangers of leakage. Simple closure of the wound of the colon, however small, is always accompanied by a risk. The decision to take such a risk must be based on experience, not ignorance. The rule that injured segments of colon should either be exteriorized or functionally excluded by a proximal colostomy is one that every surgeon should follow when he first deals with bullet wounds of the colon.

There are three basic methods of dealing with colon injured by missiles.
1. Repair by suture with or without proximal colostomy.
2. Resection with or without primary anastomosis.
3. Exteriorization of the damaged or repaired colon.

The whole colon above the lower pelvic portion is either mobile or can be readily mobilized. Injuries of these portions may, therefore, be brought onto the surface of the abdomen as a loop colostomy. A small perforation may be brought out as the apex of the loop colostomy or may be repaired and brought out in similar fashion. If the colon leaks it will leak to the outside only and when the condition has settled down the colon can be repaired and the loop returned to the abdomen. Mobilization must be sufficient to allow the colon above and below the injury to be approximated without tension. Due to the difficulties of its liquid content the right colon should **not** be exteriorized, but transverse and descending colon are readily exteriorized and this method is still very useful on occasions.

Right colon
Wounds of the right colon are not satisfactorily managed by exteriorization. The liquid nature of the faeces and the enzymatic contents cause intractable problems, with contamination of the abdominal wall and infection and in addition it is not possible to secure a satisfactory appliance. Wounds of the right colon can be managed in one of three different ways depending upon the extent of the injury to the colon and the associated visceral damage. When there is severe disruptive injury to the right colon, or when there are associated injuries to other viscera, then resection of the involved colon should be performed followed by the construction of an ileostomy and a distal mucous fistula of the colon. This is the safest and the preferred treatment for a high velocity wound of the right colon (Fig. 9.3(b)).

Resection and ileocolostomy should only be done in certain highly selected cases. It should be reserved for relatively mild injuries of the right colon in which there are no serious associated injuries to the liver, kidney, ureter or duodenum. If this procedure is performed in the

Right colon

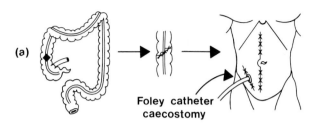

(a)

Foley catheter
caecostomy

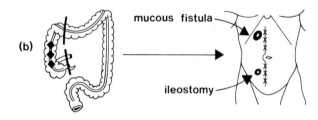

(b)

mucous fistula

ileostomy

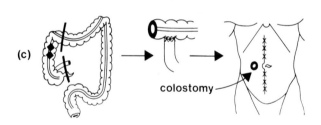

(c)

colostomy

Fig. 9.3 Right colon. Diagrammatic representation of methods of treatment of wounds of the right colon.

presence of multivisceral injury there is a significant number of anastomotic leaks which result in intra-abdominal sepsis, abscess formation and unacceptable mortality. When it is performed, the damaged segment of right colon should be resected and the continuity may be re-established by ileocolostomy (Fig. 9.3 (c)). The anastomosis is accomplished by a standard two-layer technique, preferably end-to-side, and if there is the slightest doubt, the anastomosis should be decompressed using a catheter, or by Muir's procedure.

Simple repair with or without proximal catheter caecostomy should be reserved for the uncomplicated low velocity wounds with minimal damage to the colon (Fig. 9.3 (a)).

Transverse colon

The transverse colon lends itself readily to exteriorization after missile injury (Fig. 9.4 (a)). When severe disruptive injury has occurred, resection of the involved segment is straightforward and should be followed by a functioning colostomy and distal mucous fistula (Fig. 9.4(b), 9.5). Minor wounds can be treated by repair or resection but should be protected by a proximal colostomy.

Left colon

Left colon injuries, like those of the transverse colon, can usually be exteriorized, but adequate mobilization of the colon is imperative so that there is no tension on the exteriorized loop of bowel (Fig. 9.6(a)). When there is severe disruptive injury, or a devitalized segment, then resection may be performed with end colostomy and distal mucous fistula (Fig 9.6(c)). When there are small wounds of the lower sigmoid colon which

Transverse colon

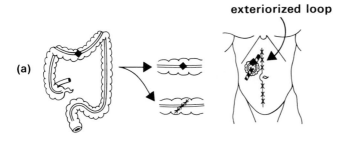

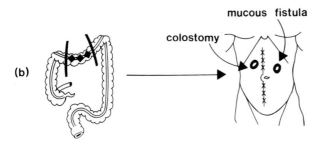

Fig. 9.4 Transverse colon. Diagrammatic representation of the methods of treatment of wounds of the transverse colon.

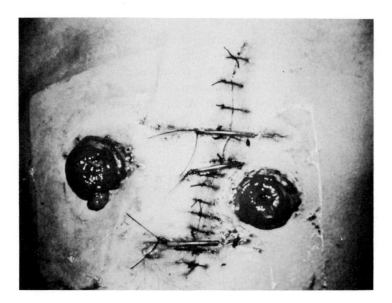

Fig. 9.5 Major wound of the transverse colon treated by resection, colostomy and mucous fistula. (Courtesy of Mr Adrian Boyd)

cannot be exteriorized, they may be closed in the standard two layers but a proximal defunctioning colostomy must be performed (Fig. 9.6(b)). When severe injury occurs to the lower sigmoid colon it may be necessary to resect the injured colon to form a proximal colostomy and to close the distal colon in two layers in the fashion of a Hartmann's operation as a blind pouch. The damaged colon, or the colostomy, should be brought out through a separate incision so placed that further contamination of the traumatic wound or the surgical incision does not take place and so that an appliance can be readily applied to the proximal stoma.

In all these severe colon wounds there is gross contamination and following operation, it is absolutely vital to establish adequate posterior dependant drainage of the paracolic gutters and subhepatic spaces.

Rectum

Wounds of the rectum have a high morbidity and mortality for they are often complicated by fractures of the pelvis, perforations of the small bowel, perforations of the bladder and damage to the urethra, major nerve injuries, and haemorrhage from blood vessels. It is most important that penetration of the rectum should be proved or excluded at the first examination. Therefore, whenever such an injury is suspected or when blood has been passed, the rectum should be examined digitally and with

Left colon

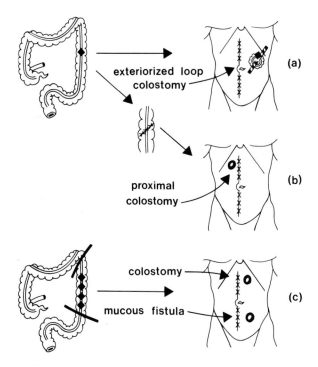

exteringized loop
colostomy

(a)

proximal
colostomy

(b)

colostomy

mucous fistula

(c)

Fig. 9.6 Diagrammatic representation of methods of treatment of wounds of the left colon.

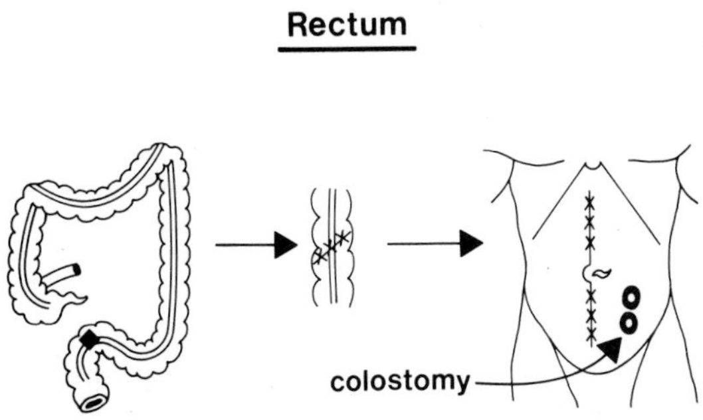

Rectum

colostomy

Fig. 9.7 Diagrammatic representation of methods of treatment of wounds of the rectum.

proctoscope and sigmoidoscope. The treatment of wounds of the rectum is by repair, thorough drainage and the formation of a defunctioning colostomy as it is most important that the faecal stream should be diverted (Fig. 9.7). The distal rectal segment should be irrigated at the time of initial surgery. Adequate drainage is vital and usually this means that the retrorectal space must be drained by drains introduced through an incision placed in the median raphe between coccyx and anus. The space between the sacrum and the rectum can then be opened up to allow excellent dependant drainage.

When defunctioning colostomy is performed it is better to divide the colon and bring each part out separately so that, on each occasion, the proximal colostomy is functioning and the distal one is a mucous fistula.

Spleen

The spleen is less often damaged than the liver due, mainly, to its smaller size but its viability and greater vascularity make it more susceptible to blows, crush injuries and blast injury. The treatment of injuries of the spleen is splenectomy. The left subphrenic space must be thoroughly drained because subphrenic infection is the most common complication following splenectomy and is usually related to injuries that have occurred to other viscera.

Pancreas

Wounds of this organ are not often met by the surgeon dealing with bullet wounds because such injuries are usually complicated due to the proximity of major vessels and are usually lethal. The pancreas must be examined at operation whenever there is a wound in the upper abdomen. Minor injuries of the pancreas, in which there is minimal contusion or laceration, should be treated simply by thorough dependant drainage through the posterior aspect of the flank. When there are more severe injuries which involve the pancreas, particularly when there is disruption of pancreatic tissue and ducts, they should be treated by resection of the distal pancreatic remnant and ligation at the proximal end of the divided pancreatic duct. The pancreatic capsule should be closed, if possible, and thorough posterior dependent drainage ensured. Wounds of the head of the pancreas should be treated by drainage alone.

Liver

The liver may be wounded by penetrating or non-penetrating injuries. In the context of bullet wounds and explosive blast injuries they may be divided into those that are caused by high velocity missiles, those caused by low velocity missiles, whether these be primary or secondary, and lastly the tertiary effects of an explosion or a missile may cause the patient to be thrown violently to the ground creating blunt, non-penetrating injuries. For the purpose of of treatment, liver wounds may be arbitrarily classified into two types according to their severity.

Low velocity fragment penetrating the liver
Such wounds usually present with slight to moderate bleeding and with limited damage to the tissues of the liver. Low velocity missile fragments and low energy blunt injuries may cause shattering of the liver parenchyma and haemorrhage of moderate to severe degree.

High velocity missiles
These will cause extensive shattering of the liver parenchyma and this is always associated with severe haemorrhage. This type of wound is a severe one and carries a high mortality. Most penetrating wounds in the region of the liver will give an obvious indication that the liver may be damaged. However, penetrating wounds of the chest from high velocity missiles can also cause extensive damage to the liver by the cavitational process. The most important clues as to the urgency of treatment comes from the knowledge as to whether the missile was of low or high velocity, in the clinical assessment of the degree of shock and in the response of the patient to resuscitation measures. High velocity missile injuries, the presence of severe shock and failure to respond rapidly to resuscitation are all indications for early operation.

Wide exposure is necessary. It is reasonable to begin the exploration through a mid-line or right paramedian abdominal incision but a thoracic extension should be made without hesitation. Damage to the left lobe can usually be managed entirely from within the abdomen whereas major damage to the right lobe can only be effectively assessed and managed surgically through a thoraco-abdominal incision. If difficulty is encountered in wounds of either side, it may usually be resolved by enlarging the incision, usually into the right thorax, since then the inferior vena cava can be approached and controlled. Splitting the sternum above the xiphisternum by extending the mid-line abdominal incision gives an extremely good exposure of the liver and is an excellent alternative approach.

Temporary control of bleeding can be achieved by packing, manual compression of the liver edges or by squeezing the structures of the portal triad with the fingers. If inflow occlusion is used, then it should be released after about ten minutes because the liver will not tolerate ischaemia for longer than this at normal temperatures. In complex parenchymal and vascular injuries inflow occlusion may be needed for longer than this and using hypothermia with oesophageal temperatures of

30–32°C occlusion can be maintained for at least 30 minutes. Peritoneal hypothermia is the most useful method under these circumstances since that can be instituted at the time of laparotomy with materials that are to be found in most operating theatres.

Definitive treatment of the liver wound
Haemostasis can be achieved by ligation of individual vessels with fine non-absorbable material supplemented by a row of interlocking through and through mattress sutures placed 2 cm back from the line of injury or proposed resection. Thick Dexon or catgut, carried on long, fine, round bodied needles should be used for these sutures. Packing must not be used for definitive haemostasis unless all other methods have failed. It has been shown that reducing the incidence of packing as definitive treatment of liver wounds and increasing the use of excision of damaged tissue and adequate drainage of the liver area, has been associated with a reduction of mortality from liver injuries. Excision of devitalized liver tissue can be done by blunt dissection through the liver beyond the margin of the damage area. The resection can be done through normal liver tissue bluntly by using an artery forceps or handle of a scalpel, or better still and more rapidly, by squeezing the tissue between the fingers so that the resistant vascular and biliary duct structures can be felt and individually ligated as they are encountered. The cut edge of the liver is secured by a line of interlocking sutures to limit any further bleeding from the parenchyma. The use of diathermy to cut the tissues is not of much value as it will not stop bleeding from the large vessels or prevent bile leakage from the bile ducts. Recent developments using *lasers* have given great hopes that their successful use in liver resections in animals may be extended to extensive liver trauma in humans. If available a laser suitable for use in an operating theatre can be used for local or extensive resections of liver tissue, and vessels up to 5 mm in diameter can be coagulated using the device. Surface damage of the remaining tissue extends to a depth of less than one millimetre. If difficulty is encountered in securing haemostasis after excision of devitalized tissue a pedicled flap of greater omentum based on its gastroepiploic blood vessels may be packed into the area and secured there. Thorough drainage, usually a sump drain, should be provided.

Most of the severe devitalizing injuries can be managed by this type of extempore resection. On occasions, however, massive injury demands formal resection of a segment or of a lobe, both to remove the devitalized tissue as part of the wound excision process and to secure control of the bleeding. Segmental resections and right or left hepatic lobectomy demand knowledge of the intrahepatic anatomy and the consequent planes for resection.

Formal resection of the liver

The anatomy of the liver should be regarded as a segmental one based upon its vascular supply and biliary drainage. Broadly speaking the segments are collected together to form the right and left lobes. These are supplied by main branches of the hepatic artery and the portal vein and the biliary drainage is to main tributaries of the hepatic duct. The ramifications of the structures of the portal triad divide the liver into fairly constant segments and on this basis the junction of the right and left lobes lies along the line drawn between the fossa of the gall bladder and the inferior vena cava. The left lobe is further divided into medial and lateral segments along the line of attachment of the ligamentum teres. The venous drainage of the liver follows a rather different arrangement for the hepatic veins within the liver lie in the intersegmental planes. There are three main hepatic veins, right, middle and left, and they all tend to have virtually no extrahepatic course and, therefore, at operation have to be approached and secured for purposes of resection in the substance of the liver itself.

Armed with such basic knowledge of the intrahepatic anatomy, it is possible to do a formal resection when it is necessary by virtue of a severe missile wound of the liver.

Right hepatic lobectomy requires a thoraco-abdominal incision along the line of the sixth or seventh rib. The diaphragm can be incised straight down to the inferior vena cava along a line passing in front of the main trunk of the phrenic nerve or alternatively around the circumference of the diaphragm, one inch from the costal margin. Both these incisions produce the least possible interference with the innervation of the diaphragm. The coronary ligament can then be incised and the liver detached from the diaphragm as far as the inferior vena cava. During this time, temporary control of bleeding from the injured liver can be obtained by digital compression of the vessels of the portal triad or by the use of a vascular clamp or an intestinal spring clamp. At the same time direct pressure by packing or with the hand can be effected on the liver itself. The right hepatic duct is identified and the right hepatic artery and right branch of the portal vein are identified and ligated. This usually produces a line of demarcation that acts as the guide to the necessary resection. This line of demarcation runs across the liver between the gall bladder fossa and the inferior vena cava. Resection for trauma should take place just to the right of this major plane by blunt dissection and this should allow preservation of the middle hepatic vein. The right hepatic vein should be secured from within the liver substance at the upper end of the resection by blunt dissection taken a little more laterally until the vein is encountered. Finally the raw surface of the liver can be left alone and the area thoroughly drained.

Left hepatic lobectomy follows a very similar procedure. The left branches or the portal triad are displayed, ligated and divided. This time the plane of resection lies to the left of the main interlobar plane. The left hepatic vein must be approached through the liver substance and secured well clear of the inferior vena cava.

Left lateral segmental resection is possible when injury is confined to the extreme left side of the liver. This segment lies to the left of the line of the ligamentum teres and resection is usually quite simple and usually only an abdominal incision is required. After mobilization of the left lobe of the liver, a line of interlocking mattress sutures can be placed just to the left of the position of the ligamentum teres. The liver is then divided by blunt dissection to the left of these sutures. Vessels and ducts that are encountered are ligated and divided separately.

Thorough abdominal drainage must be used for all liver injuries. There is little doubt that the mortality of missile wounds of the liver has been significantly reduced by the increased acceptance of drainage as an essential part of the management. Sump drains are the most effective method of peritoneal drainage and it is important that the opening through the abdominal wall must be adequate so that there is no hinderance to free drainage. Small lacerations of the liver may be treated adequately by Penrose drains down to the liver injury and also into Morrison's pouch.

Biliary decompression has been shown to reduce biliary leakage from liver lacerations but there is no need for it to be used after every injury and its use should be confined to cases of severe liver injury. T-tube drainage of the common duct should not be used routinely but it is useful for major injuries with large duct transection. In addition it offers an excellent means for later diagnostic study by cholangiography. It must always be used in association with adequate external drainage.

Vascular injuries around the porta hepatis should be repaired, where possible, according to established vascular techniques. Rarely, ligation of either portal vein or hepatic artery may have to be performed. Ligation of the latter, in particular, is poorly tolerated but has been successful in a number of cases. Injuries of the inferior vena cava and hepatic vein carry a very high mortality. Vascular isolation of the liver using inflow occlusion and vena caval occlusion around a right atrial cannula above and below the liver may be the only way of managing this problem. A subcapsular haematoma should be evacuated and the underlying damage to the parenchyma repaired. Intrahepatic haematomata are probably best treated by hepatic lobectomy.

Wound closure must be meticulous. When there has been considerable peritoneal soiling retention sutures should be used. If the entry and exit wounds are from a high velocity missile and have been used for access by extending them, then the superficial layers of the wound must be left open for delayed primary closure.

Following liver injury, particularly when resection has been done, metabolic deficiencies such as hypoglycaemia, hypoalbuminaemia and a bleeding diathesis may occur. Infection, haemobilia, secondary haemorrhage and biliary fistulae can usually be avoided by adequate treatment at the initial operation.

References and Further Reading

Artz, C. P., Bronwell, A. W. and Sako, Y. (1955). Experience in the management of abdominal and thoraco-abdominal injuries in Korea. *American Journal of Surgery*, **89**, 773–8.

Blackburn, G. and d'Abreu, A. L. (1946). Thoraco-abdominal wounds in war. *British Journal of Surgery*, **33**, 152–4.

Blackburn, G. and Rob, C. G. (1946). The abdominal wound in the field. *British Journal of Surgery*, **33**, 46–52.

Gordon-Taylor, G. (1944). Second thoughts on the abdominal surgery of total war. *British Journal of Surgery*, **32**, 247–58.

Gordon-Taylor, G. (1952). War wounds of the abdomen. *British Journal of Surgery*, War Surgery Supplement **3**, 409–522.

Haygood, F. D. and Polk, H. C. (1976). Gunshot wounds of the colon. *American Journal of Surgery*, **131**, 213–18.

Kirkpatrick, J. R. (1977). Injuries of the colon. In Symposium on trauma. *Surgical Clinics of North America*, **57**, 67–76

Madding, G. F. Lim, R. C. and Kennedy, P. A. (1977). Hepatic and vena caval injuries. *Surgical Clinics of North America*, **57** (2), 275–89.

Nwafo, D. C. (1980). Selective primary suture of the battle injured colon: an experience of the Nigerian Civil War. *British Journal of Surgery*, **67**, 195–7.

Parks, T. G. (1979). Surgical management of gunshot injuries of the large intestine. *Journal of the Royal Society of Medicine*, **72**, 412–14.

Stevenson, H. M. and Wilson, W. (1975). Gunshot wounds of the trunk. *British Medical Journal*, **1**, 728–30.

Wallace, C. (1918). *War Surgery of the Abdomen*. J. and A. Churchill, London.

10

Chest

Any wound of the chest has two results. The first is the damage that is done by the penetrating missile, whether it be primary or secondary, and the second is the effect that any wound or injury may have on disturbing pulmonary and cardiac functions and which if they are not promptly corrected may well prove fatal. All chest wounds must be regarded as potentially serious no matter how small the wound and however good the patient's condition may appear when first seen (Fig. 10.1).

Direct damage to the chest from penetrating wounds may involve the chest wall, the lungs, the oesophagus and mediastinal contents, the

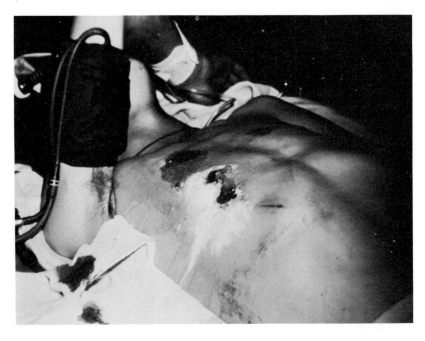

Fig. 10.1 Two high velocity bullet wounds of the right side of the chest. The patient made uncomplicated, rapid recovery.

heart and the diaphragm. As was shown in Part 1 on Mechanism of Injury, the lung itsef is remarkably resistant to damage from penetrating missiles whereas the heart and mediastinal contents are much more susceptible. Chest wounds are often complicated by damage to the abdomen or to the neck.

In pure blast injuries and occasionally with crushing injuries there may be extensive internal damage with no obvious external signs of this.

Complications

Many of the complications of these injuries are related to mechanical changes which often have profound physiological effects. These complications may be considered under the following headings:
Pneumothorax
Tension pneumothorax
Haemothorax
Subcutaneous emphysema
Flail chest
Cardiac tamponade
Explosive blast injuries
Thoracoabdominal wounds

Pneumothorax
In all penetrating wounds of the lungs some air inevitably escapes into the pleural space (Fig. 10.2). The reduction in the volume of the lung and therefore the reduction in vital capacity is proportional to the size of the pneumothorax. A small pneumothorax would usually be absorbed over a few days. Its presence has little effect and there is usually no need of active treatment. A larger pneumothorax can usually be diagnosed clinically by the reduction of chest movements, hyper-resonance and reduced breath sounds on the affected side. The diagnosis is usually confirmed by chest radiograph (Fig. 10.3). An open pneumothorax occurs when wounds of the chest wall allow air to enter and leave the pleural space during respiration. Such wounds are called 'sucking wounds of the chest' because of the sound made as the air passes in and out of the chest cavity bubbling through any blood that is present. The lung on the wounded side collapses away from the chest wall and during inspiration air is drawn from this lung into the opposite lung and the mediastinum is therefore displaced towards the undamaged side. During expiration air is blown from the sound lung into the damaged lung and the mediastinum is displaced towards the wounded side; thus, paradoxical ventilation occurs and the quantity of air which reaches the lung is less than normal and it contains an excess of carbon dioxide and a reduced

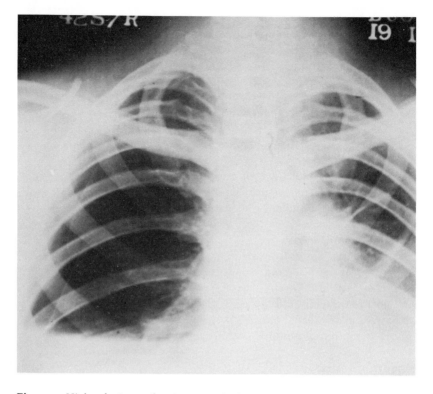

Fig. 10.2 High velocity perforating wound of the right lung. This has created a small pneumothorax and the edge of the collapsed lung can be seen. There is also a moderate haemothorax.

proportion of oxygen. Dyspnoea and cyanosis increase, the mediastinal to and from movements become more and more violent and eventually this impedes the venous return from the great vessels to the heart so that the cardiac output is diminished. The sucking wound of the chest is one of the major emergencies that must be dealt with immediately. It is second only to the maintenance of the clear airway and its treatment must be taught to all medical personnel and also first-aiders. The first-aid treatment is to close the sucking wound of the chest by the application of a large dressing which blocks the passage of air in and out of the wound from the pleural cavity; thus the mechanical disturbance is reduced and the undamaged lung is allowed to function more favourably.

Tension pneumothorax

In some penetrating wounds the leak from the lung or the chest wall may be valvular so that air is allowed to enter into the pleural space but

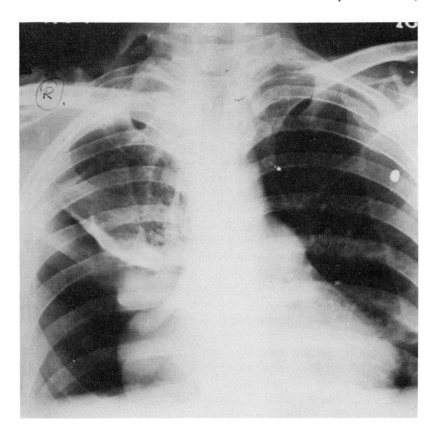

Fig. 10.3 High velocity perforating wound of the right side of the chest. In this case there is a large pneumothorax and the lung has collapsed down, particularly in the lower lobe. There is a small haemothorax and the fluid level is clearly shown.

not leave it. This means that the pneumothorax increases in volume and pressure, compresses the wounded lung, displaces the mediastinum to the opposite side and compresses the normal lung. The tension pneumothorax is recognized by the reduced costal movements, hyper-resonance to percussion and reduction of breath sounds together with the shift of the trachea and the apex beat of the heart to the opposite side. These changes are usually accompanied by dyspnoea, cyanosis and pallor. This, again, is a most urgent emergency. The tension pneumothorax must be relieved and the pressure reduced otherwise the condition will deteriorate rapidly and the patient may die within minutes. Relief is usually obtained by passing a wide bore needle through the chest wall into the pleural cavity allowing the air under pressure to escape. If available a chest catheter on a rigid introducer such as the Argyle is used and this can be connected to a Heimlich one-way valve for effective treatment of the pneumothorax once the pressure has been reduced. The cathether can be connected to an underwater seal for definitive treatment at leisure, because the emergency is over.

Haemothorax

After chest wounds, whether they be open or closed, blood may accumulate in the pleural space and it can originate from the lung, mediastinal contents and the chest wall. Bleeding from the lung is usually slow and ceases spontaneously whereas bleeding from the hilar or systemic vessels is sometimes massive. The volume of the haemothorax is later increased by effusion into it from the pleura so that the haemoglobin content is, in many cases, about half that of the circulating blood. On clinical examination, the physical signs are those of a pleural effusion combined with those of loss of blood. The trachea and mediastinum may be displaced to the side opposite that of injury and the shift of the apex beat of the heart can be a useful indicator, particularly with shift to the left. If the haemothorax, when first seen, is large enough to cause displacement of the mediastinum and dyspnoea, this is usually an indication that there is continued bleeding from a parietal or mediastinal blood vessel as opposed to bleeding from the lung itself. The contents of a haemothorax would usually remain liquid but with the passage of time a variable degree of clotting occurs. Fibrin is deposited from blood, particularly on the pleural surface of the lung and if the haemothorax persists and is not effectively drained the fibrin may become organized to form a thick cortex covering the lung and preventing its re-expansion. The more quickly a significant haemothorax is drained the less chance there is of later decortication of the lung being required (Figs. 10.2 and 10.3).

Subcutaneous emphysema

With any penetrating chest wound and in some closed chest injuries, air may escape from a pneumothorax into the soft tissues of the chest wall and crepitus can be readily demonstrated. With a tension pneumothorax considerable quantities of air may be forced into the parietal tissues and the emphysema is much more extensive. If the surgical emphysema begins on the chest wall and then spreads up into the neck and the face and downwards across the abdomen the likelihood is that the emphysema is not of itself dangerous and in the course of time the air will absorb and the inflated tissues will return to normal. When surgical emphysema is first detected in the region of the suprasternal notch, the supraclavicular areas, or is largely confined to the neck, then it suggests that the leakage is coming from the trachea, the oesophagus or a major bronchus and that the escaped air has passed up the mediastinum to appear in the neck. This physical sign may be of great importance in the detection and treatment of such injuries.

Flail chest
When a segment of the chest wall loses its rigidity because of double fractures occurring in several ribs or in multiple fractures involving ribs and sternum, the effects produced are similar to those already described in the sucking wound of the chest. The mobile section of the chest wall moves in paradoxical fashion being drawn inwards during inspiration and blown outwards during expiration. This is exactly the reverse of the movement normally found in respiration. The air in the lungs tends to move from one to another, the mediastinum shifts to and fro in pendulum fashion and the patient loses the ability to cough effectively and expel retained secretions. As in sucking wounds of the chest, paradoxical movement and all its consequences can be reduced by the application of a large, firm dressing which supports the flail segment of the chest.

Cardiac tamponade
Wounds of the heart are commonly fatal, but occasionally with a low velocity penetrating injury or in a blunt injury the pericardium remains intact and the injury may be followed by bleeding which fills and distends the pericardium. As the pressure increases inside the pericardium, obstruction of the venous return to the heart occurs and this prevents normal atrial filling. Cardiac tamponade can usually be recognized by the characteristic distension of the veins of the neck, the weak, thready pulse, associated with a narrow pulse pressure. If the cardiac tamponade is not relieved as a matter of urgency death from circulatory failure may follow. Emergency drainage of the blood in the pericardium can usually be done by aspirating the pericardium with a needle.

Explosive blast injuries
Injuries to the lung from the blast wave at some distance from an explosive weapon must always be considered when the patient has been exposed to the risk of such damage. In pure blast injuries there are usually no external signs of damage and the first signs are commonly delayed for as long as 24 hours or more before they become obvious. These signs include restlessness, dyspnoea, haemoptysis, chest pain and later cyanosis and reduced Po_2 and a raised Pco_2. If emergency treatment is required endotracheal intubation and positive pressure ventilation is necessary. A chest radiograph reveals the characteristic appearance of extensive lung mottling. Severe blast injuries of the lung are commonly associated with

pneumothoraces or haemopneumothoraces and in this case the emergency treatment involves the insertion of bilateral intercostal catheters and in addition, in some cases, endotracheal intubation and positive pressure ventilation.

Thoracoabdominal wounds
Both abdomen and thorax may be damaged from a penetrating missile entering the other cavity. Thoracoabdominal wounds occur more frequently than abdominothoracic ones and have a better prognosis. Wounds of the right side have a better prognosis than those of the left. In general thoracoabdominal wounds are classified separately because they have a higher mortality than chest wounds alone.

Principles of treatment

The treatment of penetrating chest wounds follows the well established principles of wounds of soft tissues and in addition the application of special principles which have been derived from knowledge of respiratory and circulatory disorders.

Normal intrathoracic pressures
It is essential that pleural and pericardial spaces should be kept empty and that their normal pressures should be maintained. This requires release of the tension pneumothorax, aspiration of the pericardium for cardiac tamponade, the closure of an open pneumothorax, stabilization of the stove-in chest and drainage of a large pneumothorax or haemothorax.

Clearance of bronchial tree
This must be kept free of retained blood, bronchial secretions and foreign material. Clearance of the bronchi can be made more effective by utilizing the methods described in the preceding paragraph, in the relief of pain to allow adequate and productive coughing by postural drainage and finally by tracheal and bronchoscopic aspiration. Tracheostomy may be required to reduce the ventilatory dead space and airways resistance and it will also facilitate frequent aspiration of bronchial secretions.

Control and replacement of blood loss
Bleeding from penetrating chest wounds is usually from intercostal or internal mammary vessels; the lung itself does not usually bleed much. Massive haemorrhage from major pulmonary vessels or the vessels in the mediastinum usually causes early death before medical help can be

given. The basis of treatment is the withdrawal of the blood-stained effusion from the pleural space and replacement of the estimated and measured blood lost. The measurement of blood draining from the pleural cavity must be carefully recorded for this value is critical in determining the need or otherwise for emergency surgery to control the haemorrhage.

First-aid treatment of chest wounds

The perforating or penetrating wound of the chest without any complications requires little direct attention. Haemoptysis is common and this should be explained to the patient who should be reassured before evacuation. The open sucking wounds of the chest must be closed immediately. Such a wound may be fatal because of the physiological effects on the respiratory and circulatory system when paradoxical respiration occurs as explained under the section on Pneumothorax. This is accomplished by firmly packing the open wound with an occlusive dressing. This dressing is more effective if it is wet or impregnated with Vaseline type material. The dressing can usually be kept in place with strapping but a few sutures may, occasionally, be necessary. A tension pneumothorax may occur after successful occlusion of a sucking chest wound and in this case a chest tube must be inserted. Small segments of flail chest may be temporarily stabilized by a dressing firmly strapped over the mobile segment of the chest wall. The strapping must be applied only over the involved area of the chest wall so that it does not unduly limit the function of the remaining part of the chest. If there is evidence of cardiac tamponade, the pericardium must be aspirated. A needle should be inserted in the angle between the xiphisternum and the costal margin and should be passed upwards and backwards at an angle of 45° into the pericardial sac. This aspiration may be repeated until such time as emergency thoracotomy can be performed.

Management in the casualty department

Once again the most essential treatment of penetrating or closed chest injuries is based on a system of priorities and an immediate check must be made on the airway, whether there is clinical evidence of pneumothorax or haemothorax, shift of the mediastinum, cardiac tamponade or signs of continued external or internal thoracic bleeding. A chest x-ray is done at this stage, but remember that the clinical evidence of tension pneumothorax, a sucking wound of the chest or bilateral chest involvement must take priority over the chest x-ray and treatment should be instituted immediately.

Control of the airway

This may be difficult in a patient with an injury to the upper airway, in the deeply comatose patient or those with severe flail chest. Endotracheal intubation is preferred initially and this can be followed if necessary, by a tracheostomy done as an elective procedure at a later time.

Closed tube thoracostomy

If clinical examination reveals signs of blood or air in the pleural space an intercostal drainage tube should be inserted immediately. Recent war experience has proven that early and adequate evacuation of the pleural space by large chest tubes is essential. A large bore chest tube, for example an Argyle 32 Fr should be inserted, in an upwards direction, through the lateral, lower chest wall in the mid-axillary line for removal of blood and fluid. A similar tube should be placed in the second interspace anteriorly for the removal of air from any significant pneumothorax. Both tubes may be connected initially to Heimlich one-way valves and thence, in a closed system, to drainage bags. Underwater seal suction drainage should be applied to both drains as soon as practicable. A chest radiograph should be taken afterwards to confirm location of the tube, the evacuation of the pleural space and to locate any foreign bodies. The tubes may be removed when there is no longer any evidence of air leak and when fluid and air are no longer present.

Aspiration of the pericardial sac may have to be repeated if there is continued evidence of cardiac tamponade and this is used as a preliminary to thoracotomy.

There is no necessity to do an open thoracotomy routinely on all wounds of the chest. Thoracotomy may be required for the following indications:

Continued intrathoracic bleeding

Abdominothoracic injury with suspected intraperitoneal injury

Massive continuing air leak

Injury to the mediastinal contents such as the great vessels, trachea or oesophagus

Cardiac tamponade or cardiac wounds

Sucking wounds of the chest

Large wounds of the chest wall, particularly those where there is a defect.

Under ideal conditions where there are adequate facilities and staff and no excess of casualties to be dealt with it may be preferable to deal with all known high velocity penetrating wounds of the chest by formal thoracotomy. However, it is emphasized that provided that closed tube thoracostomy is initiated early and adequate drainage of blood from the pleural cavity is obtained, then there is no need to do thoracotomy on all penetrating chest wounds. There is evidence, however, that thoracotomy in all cases, where possible, does reduce the incidence of complications due to deposition of fibrin from poorly drained pleural cavities and reduces the incidence of later decortication of affected lungs.

The major indication for thoracotomy used in wartime and by those surgeons who are experienced in the management of penetrating missile wounds is continued or massive intrathoracic bleeding. The next most frequent indication for thoracotomy is that of the large defect of the chest wall. Air leak and mediastinal injuries are uncommon indications for thoracotomy. General anaesthesia with endotracheal intubation and controlled positive pressure respiration is required in all cases.

Operation

When thoracotomy is required the majority of chest wounds may be dealt with through a standard posterior lateral thoracotomy through the sixth interspace or the bed of the sixth rib. This approach will give good access to all the intrathoracic organs from the same side. Blood and blood clot are removed from the pleural space and the bleeding vessel must be found and secured. Such bleeding usually comes from an intercostal artery or the internal mammary artery. Bleeding from the lung usually ends once the lung has been inflated and comes into contact with the chest wall. In some lung wounds ligation of bleeding vessels and oversewing of a small segment of lung may be necessary. Pulmonary resection is seldom necessary and as shown in the Chapter 2 on Ballistics, the lung has remarkable powers of recovery. On occasions, however, when a segmental or lobar bronchus has been damaged, resection of the appropriate lobe may be necessary. In other cases most leaks can be closed by ligation of small and suture of larger bronchi. All fragments of bone and all foreign bodies in the pleura or lung should be removed if they are readily accessible. Every effort should be made to remove accessible clothing, fragments and other organic debris but no prolonged search should be made for inaccessible metallic foreign bodies which may have been demonstrated on the radiographs. The wound of the chest wall must be treated in exactly the same fashion as for all soft tissue wounds, there must be adequate excision of all damaged tissue in all layers of the chest. Skin requires minimal excision, damaged muscle and fascia must be removed until healthy tissue is reached, small shattered fragments of ribs should be removed and the injured rib ends nibbled away until they are smooth in order to prevent damage to the pleura or lung at a later stage. The pleura should then be closed if possible, usually taking a layer of muscle to ensure an airtight closure and the remainder of the wounds should be left open for delayed primary closure. If the defect in the chest wall is large, making such closure difficult or impossible, then sliding grafts of the muscle of the chest wall must be made to close the defect and such defects may sometimes require the use of a synthetic mesh as a last resort.

Wounds of the heart and proximal great vessels are best approached through a median sternotomy and this may need to be extended into the neck in order to get control of the major vessels in the root of the neck by turning a flap. Suspicion of injury to the vascular structures of the mediastinum requires early exploration and access to the great vessels in the chest may be rapidly obtained by an anterior thoracotomy in the third interspace on the involved side which permits control of the bleeding. This can later be extended into a formal sternotomy. If thoracotomy has been done for cardiac tamponade the pericardium should be opened from apex to base; harmorrhage can be controlled by digital pressure whilst closing the cardiac wound. The pericardium should only be loosely closed so that any fluid can escape freely into the pleural space rather than be retained in the pericardium. Oesophageal perforations should be closed by direct suture paying particular attention to closing the tough grey mucosal layer as this is the secure layer of the oesophagus.

Thoracoabdominal wounds

Thoracic wounds will quite often produce abdominal physical signs even though the abdominal cavity has not been penetrated; nevertheless, one should always remember that a penetrating wound of the chest or abdomen can involve the other cavity and this is particularly true of high velocity missiles. Some guidance may be given by the entry and exit wounds and the possible course of the missile, particularly when this is taken into conjunction with the location of foreign bodies demonstrated on the radiograph. Remember how high the diaphragm rises into the chest during expiration and how deep are the costophrenic sulci particularly laterally and posteriorly. Most of these wounds, by the nature of the cavitational process, are grossly contaminated and the temptation to use a thoraco-abdominal approach as for elective cold surgery should be resisted. The majority of thoracoabdominal wounds can be managed by intercostal tube drainage of the pleural space and laparotomy to treat the abdominal injuries and repair the diaphragm from below. Similarly, an abdominothoracic injury may well be better treated by a thorough laparotomy and treatment of all intra-abdominal injuries and occasionally a small separate thoracotomy is required to repair the right side of the diaphragm when this is not possible from below. If this thoracic wound is extensive it will require thorough wound excision, closure of the pleura with adequate drainage of the pleural space and delayed primary closure of the superficial parts of the wound. In wartime about 25 per cent of thoracic wounds also involve the abdominal cavity and in general by virtue of this involvement the patient's prognosis is worse than if the chest alone was involved.

Management after operation

Scrupulous attention to detail must be emphasized in the management after operation. Chest tubes must be constantly checked to see if they are patent, that underwater seals are working and that radiographs confirm the position of the tubes and the expansion of the lungs and the removal of any intrapleural fluid. There must be adequate pulmonary ventilation and the persistent removal of tracheobronchial secretions by coughing, suction and bronchoscopic aspiration as necessary. The patient may well need to be placed on assisted ventilation through either the endotracheal tube or a tracheostomy. Once blood and other fluids have been replaced, the administration of further intravenous fluid should be cautious during the period after operation because of the possible aggravation of post-traumatic pulmonary insufficiency. If hypoxaemia develops or there is evidence of pulmonary oedema even greater care should be given on fluid administration and diuretics will need to be used. Such cases are best managed in an intensive care unit specially equipped for the intensive respiratory management that is required.

References and Further Reading

Amato, J. J., Billy, L. J., Gruber, R. P. and Rich, N. M. (1974). Temporary cavitation in high velocity pulmonary missile injury. *Annals of Thoracic Surgery*, **18**, 565–70.
Brewer, L. A. (1969). Wounds of the chest in war and peace. *Annals of Thoracic Surgery*, **1**, 387–408.
Daniel, R. A. (1944). Bullet wounds of the lungs – An experimental study. *Surgery*, **15**, 774–82.
De Muth, W. E. (1968). High velocity bullet wounds of the thorax. *American Journal of Surgery*, **115**, 616–25.
Ferguson, D. G. and Stevenson, H. M. (1978). A review of 158 gunshot wounds to the chest. *British Journal of Surgery*, **65**, 845–7.
Glass, J. L. (1969). Treatment of chest injuries in Vietnam. *American Surgeon*, **35**, 227–8.
Gordon-Taylor, G. (1952). War wounds of the chest. *British Journal of Surgery*, War Surgery Supplement, **3**, 381–408.
McNamara, J. J. *et al.* (1970). Thoracic injuries in combat casualties in Vietnam. *Annals of Thoracic Surgery*, **10**, 389–401.

II

Neck

Wounds of the neck are frequently complicated because of the number of vital structures within this transitional area. They are frequently Priority 1 emergencies and they carry a relatively high mortality. Any injury of the neck is commonly associated with asphyxiation from an impaired airway and severe haemorrhage from the major vessels that run through the neck. Because so many structures run close together in a very limited area available, many systems can be injured by the same missile; e.g. there could be involvement of the oesophagus, the trachea or larynx and the vessels in the neck, all at the same time. Any involvement of the oropharynx or oesophagus may allow bacterial contamination of the mediastinum. All neck wounds must be managed by prime attention to the airway and control of bleeding, adequate incisions to give generous exposure and careful wound excision followed by thorough wound drainage. In an emergency situation, the airway must be controlled, usually by the use of an endotracheal tube and when there is a laryngeal injury this may well be one of the few indications for emergency tracheostomy.

Wounds of the larynx and trachea

All injuries of the trachea and larynx are potentially serious. The diagnosis should be confirmed by laryngoscopy or bronchoscopy which should be readily performed when there is the slightest suspicion of any injury. Sometimes the injury is apparent, at others it may be occult and a high index of suspicion is required to diagnose the injury. These examinations may commonly be done at the time that control of the airway is gained and at which time an endotracheal tube may be inserted. Even if emergency tracheostomy is required because of severe injuries to the larynx or hypopharynx the laryngeal injuries must nevertheless be treated, otherwise subsequent serious loss of function will be caused which may be prevented by early diagnosis and treatment.

These wounds commonly cause asphyxia and dyspnoea. The asphyxia, provided the airway is otherwise undamaged, is an indication of laryngotracheal injury. The obstruction may be caused by actual destruction of part of the larynx, fragments of which may physically block the lumen of the trachea, by haemorrhage from the injuries which blocks the airway with blood clot, or by laryngotracheal oedema caused by the missile injury. Dyspnoea may occur from obvious injuries to the larynx or trachea but lesser degrees may be caused by injuries which can only be found by careful examination. If injury is suspected the patient must be examined and note taken of any haemoptysis, dysphagia, excessive mobility of the larynx, dysphonia or the presence of a laryngeal type cough. Radiographic examination of the larynx and tracheal cartilages and laryngoscopy are of diagnostic value. Retropharyngeal swelling may be detected on direct physical examination or may be revealed by a soft tissue radiograph. Also on these radiographs, narrowing of the air column by a soft tissue mass may be a pointer to this diagnosis. Lastly subcutaneous emphysema of the face and neck may occur whenever there has been an injury to the larynx or trachea.

At operation, once the airway is fully under control and general anaesthesia has been obtained, careful and conservative excision of the damaged tissues following laryngotracheal injuries must be done. Following the excision of the wound, the fragmented larynx or trachea should be brought into anatomical alignment and an intraluminal stent used to maintain the position. It is important to avoid later laryngeal or tracheal stenosis from excessive removal of tissue, particularly the cartilage and the mucosa. At this time great care must be taken to identify any associated wounds of the adjacent structures, particularly the oesophagus and the major vessels.

Wounds of the pharynx and oesophagus

These structures are equally involved with the larynx and trachea and blood vessels in any injuries of the neck. Whenever they have been damaged, there is a definite risk of contamination of the fascial planes of the neck and the mediastinum. Any penetrating injury of the neck must be considered to have the potential of damaging the pharynx and oesophagus. Soft tissue radiographs may be useful as can endoscopy of the pharynx and oesophagus and the use of radiopaque contrast media. All such wounds must be explored, any damage must be identified, the damaged tissue must be excised and the lacerations of the mucosa and muscularis of the pharynx and oesophagus closed. If possible a double layer closure of the defects is the treatment of choice but the greatest attention should be paid to closing the tough mucosal layer. External drainage is imperative.

Vascular injuries of the neck

The neck, together with the heart and head, is one of the favourite aiming points for assassination by snipers. Many injuries of the major neck and mediastinal vascular structures are fatal. Any suspicion of injury to the vascular structure of the neck requires early exploration. Access to the great vessels in the chest is attained by an anterior thoracotomy in the third interspace on the involved side and this allows rapid control of the major vessels. A flap can then be turned by extending to a median sternotomy with resection of the medial aspect of the clavicle. The mortality from uncontrolled haemorrhage is second only to asphyxiation in injuries of the neck and, therefore, the control of the airway and early haemostasis are the two imperative steps of the management of neck injuries. Sometimes serious vascular injury can be hidden because the haemorrhage takes place into the deep fascial compartments of the neck. This may allow some slowing of the rate of bleeding but eventually this causes an enlarging haematoma which encroaches upon the airway. All explorations of the neck should involve an approach which gives early control of the upper and lower end of the carotid and internal jugular systems. After wound excision, if an artery has been damaged, lateral repair or an end-to-end anastomosis is preferred but if this is impossible, autogenous vein graft must be used to bridge an arterial defect. The use of an internal or external shunt to maintain cerebral circulation during repair is preferable. Remember that arteries can be damaged by the shock waves and cavitation so that there is cessation of blood flow even though the vessel is in continuity. This is due to the damage to the intima which usually causes an intimal flap and thrombosis. This can only be ascertained and treated by arteriotomy. If there are any associated nerve injuries these should be identified, recorded and marked. They should not be treated primarily but by delayed primary suture. High velocity missile wounds of the neck whose track passes close to the vertebral column may well cause spinal cord injury without actual damage to the cord with resultant quadriplegia.

References and Further Reading

Fitchett, V. H., Pomerantz, M., Butsch, D. W. and Eiseman, B. (1969). Penetrating wounds of the neck – a military and civilian experience. *Archives of Surgery, Chicago*, **99**, 307–14.

Jones, R. F., Terrell, J. C. and Salyer, K. E. (1967). Penetrating wounds of the neck. *Journal of Trauma*, **7**, 228–37.

McInnis, W. D., Crutz, A. B. and Austu, B. (1975). Penetrating injuries to the neck. *American Journal of Surgery*, **130,** 416–20.

Sankaran, S. and Walt, A. J. (1977). Penetrating wounds of the neck. *Surgical Clinics of North America*, **57** (1), 139–50.

12

Brain and spinal cord

Brain

Open wounds of the brain are caused by penetrating missiles, whether they be bullets or fragments from explosive devices. Closed injuries usually occur when the body is knocked over by the energy transfer from the missile or blast wave and strikes some part of the surrounding environment. This can cause closed head or spinal injuries similar to those caused in road traffic or industrial accidents.

Localized brain damage is caused by sharp impact from a stone, bottle or hand held weapons. The essential lesion is a compound depressed fracture of the skull and the damage is confined to the brain tissue which lies immediately below the fracture and the patient often remains fully conscious.

Penetrating missile wounds of the head, however, produce signs both of localized and of generalized brain damage.

The damage caused by a missile depends very much upon the amount of energy which it transfers to the tissues and the rate at which it transfers such energy. As was shown in Chapter 2 on Ballistics, the greater the velocity of the missile the more energy will be transferred to the tissues and the more the damage that will be caused. On the whole a low velocity fragment causes much less damage than a high velocity missile and the damage tends to be more localized; thus it is most important to know the velocity of the missile in order that an estimate can be made of the likely damage and the patient's prognosis.

Most accounts of penetrating cerebral missile injuries comes from experience in war-time and the major wars have been the stimulus to great improvements in the management of such penetrating missile wounds.

In World War II, in Korea and in Vietnam, over 80 per cent of the head wounds were caused by metallic fragments from mines, shells, rockets and bombs; bullet wounds only accounted for the remaining 15–20 per cent. In the Arab–Israeli war in 1973, metallic fragments were, again, responsible for the vast majority of the injuries. Head wounds caused by metallic fragments carry a much lower mortality than those caused by bullets. Head injuries caused by civil disturbance present a very

138

different picture, for the vast majority of penetrating brain wounds are due to bullets and a high proportion of these are normally caused by low velocity bullets from hand guns. In Northern Ireland less than 10 per cent of all head wounds result from explosion due to the type of explosive devices that are used and there has been an increasing severity of wound related directly to the increasing use of rifle bullets.

The brain damage depends not only upon the energy of the missile but on the angle at which it strikes the head. A tangential blow will cause a 'gutter' fracture and bone fragments are sent off as secondary missiles to be driven deeply into the brain. If the missile strikes more at right angles to the skull then the missile may traverse the brain in the line of its travel. A low velocity fragment may be regarded as coring out its path through the brain tissue and may well have not enough energy to penetrate the far side of the skull and the fragments are often retained. A high velocity fragment on the other hand, such as a rifle bullet, will usually go right through the skull causing gross damage to the brain by virtue of the cavitation effect, in which the brain is used as the mechanism to fracture the skull from the inside. There is usually extensive fracturing of the skull. Bone fragments are sent off as secondary missiles deep into the remaining parts of the brain.

Following penetrating craniocerebral trauma a varying volume of brain and meninges are destroyed, either directly by a low velocity missile or by the cavitational effects of high velocity missiles. The cells surrounding this damaged tissue becomes oedematous, cause the brain to swell and the intracranial pressure will rise. This in turn damages further cells and the cycle is repeated. Metabolites from sick cells further aggravate the situation.

Anoxaemia or hypercarbia from whatever cause will cause increasing cerebral oedema and hypercarbia will increase cerebral blood volume and thereby raise intracranial pressure.

Little can be done about the original brain injury but something can be done about reducing the subsequent damage described above. The most common source of this damage is inadequate airway care, especially partial obstruction by tongue or vomit. Even a slight increase in blood CO_2 levels can increase intracranial pressure and can cause a deterioration in cerebral blood flow. The deliberate reduction of CO_2 levels by controlled hyperventilation increases blood flow through impoverished areas of the brain.

First-aid

The first-aid treatment of such injuries is to maintain the airway by intubation if necessary and to evacuate the patient rapidly to a neurosurgical unit. Rapid evacuation is important for you must remember that about half the deaths from missile wounds of the head occur within six hours.

In a brief clinical examination, the level of consciousness, the state of the pupils and the reaction of the limbs are recorded and any other associated injuries are assessed. Patients who are alert on admission have a good prognosis with a 90 per cent chance survival. Of patients who are drowsy on admission, about 60 per cent survive; of those who are unconscious but react to painful stimuli, about 20 per cent survive and of those admitted in coma, one would expect no survivors. Those who have fixed dilated pupils have an extremely poor prognosis. Patients who have severe penetrating head injuries should be intubated immediately, if necessary using intravenous diazepam or pancuronium. It has been shown that intubation followed by controlled hyperventilation provides the best way to reduce the raised intracranial pressure. The use of a pressure transducer introduced through the wound between the dura and the skull has demonstrated the beneficial effect of controlled hyperventilation. The ventilation lowers the central venous pressure which reduces engorgement of the intracranial venous system, and it also allows the blood gas levels to be controlled at predetermined levels. Reduction of the Pco_2 level to 30–35 mm of mercury by hyperventilation encourages cerebral vasoconstriction thereby reducing the volume of the brain.

Associated injuries must be evaluated in order to obtain the correct order in which to treat the cerebral wounds. Even with a pure penetrating head injury it may be necessary to replace large quantities of blood, for severe haemorrhage commonly occurs from missile wounds of the brain. Resuscitation should be vigorous, antibiotics and steroids should be started. Once the patient has been intubated and resuscitated then he can be taken to the theatre via the x-ray Department where skull x-rays should be taken. The patient is fit, at this stage, to be transferred to another hospital where a neurosurgical facility is situated. All severe penetrating head wounds require this treatment before moving, whereas minor injuries, particularly those with low velocity bullets or fragments and who have no impairment of vital signs, may be moved without too much risk of deterioration of their condition.

Operation
The aims of surgery in gunshot wounds of the brain are:
1. To arrest haemorrhage and evacuate intracerebral haematoma.
2. To remove bone and metal fragments and to excise damaged tissue in order to combat infection.
3. To repair the dura, provide adequate scalp cover and later on to restore the contour of the skull.

Volatile anaesthetic agents should not be used as they increase intracranial pressure. The head wound is inspected and the head thoroughly shaved, cautious palpation of the extent and depth of the wound with the sterile gloved finger provides useful information regarding its extent. Taken in conjunction with the knowledge of the type of missile and the x-ray changes, a reasonably accurate assessment of the likely course of the missile and the damage to be expected can be made. The operation is carried out in the following steps:

Scalp
Skin, as always, is remarkably viable and only the minimal amount of devitalized and contaminated skin edge should be removed together with any superficial foreign bodies.

Skull
It is essential that any contaminated edges of bone should be removed as otherwise a chronic infection will ensue. Only damaged and grossly contaminated pericranium need be excised. Inspection of the damaged brain may well require wide exposure which is usually gained by reflecting a semicircular skull flap or removing some of the bone surrounding the entry and exit wound. Burr holes should be placed in intact bone close to the area of damage and the bone nibbled away by rongeurs towards the area of contamination.

Dura
The margin of normal dura should be exposed and only minimal excision of damaged dural edge is required.

Brain
Dead and damaged brain tissue must be removed by irrigation with physiological saline and gentle low pressure suction. All devitalized brain, blood clots, bone fragments and foreign bodies should be removed. It is most important that this part of the operation be done meticulously and that this first excision of the wounds should be the only one. The removal of metallic foreign bodies is not so crucial as is the removal of bone fragments. If this operation is done well there will be a low incidence of intracerebral abscesses and this is an indication of the situation in which the operation takes place and the skill and experience of the neurosurgeon involved. On many occasions there is no requirement to remove the bullet that has caused the damage and in Belfast fewer than half the bullets lodged in the brain have been removed. Thorough exploration of the wound and escision of the damaged tissues may extend as far as the ventricle or the mid-line.

Closure

Closure of the dura after the damaged brain has been thoroughly excized is regarded by most neurosurgeons, experienced in penetrating missile wounds, as essential. Closure of the dura may be obtained primarily, and if this is not possible it should be done using pericranium, temporalis fascia, galea or fascia lata. Full thickness accurate closure of the scalp is essential even if this demands rotation of a skin flap with closure of the secondary scalp defect by skin graft.

Care after operation

Radiography may indicate retained bone fragments if the wound excision has been inadequate and where possible further operation should be performed shortly, because such retained bone fragments are an indication of the incomplete nature of the operation and will usually lead to brain abscess. All patients with severe gunshot wounds of the head should continue with controlled ventilation for two or three days after operation in order to regulate their blood gases and to lower the central venous pressure. Tangenital wounds of the skull require special care because although they may appear to be minor these wounds frequently show severe damage of the brain beneath the apparently intact covering and should be treated energetically. The tangential wound of the high velocity missile always causes severe damage to the brain out of all proportion to the appearance. Compound depressed fractures resulting from such tangential wounds are best treated by craniectomy rather than by simple elevation. The dura and the brain must be inspected and, if necessary, opened. If the underlying cortex has been damaged then it must be excised in the usual way. Remember the cavitation effect of a tangential wound from a high velocity missile is the mechanism by which this damage occurs, and what may be apparently a near miss of the brain just grazing the bone, may in fact have quite severe brain involvement.

Prognosis

This is good in patients not deeply unconscious, who respond to simple commands and who do not develop signs of deterioration. The prognosis is poor in patients who are comatose and particularly if they have fixed dilated pupils. In war, when the majority of injuries are caused by fragments, many of these are low velocity and, therefore, the overall mortality is of the order of 30 per cent. In Northern Ireland where nearly 95 per cent of the penetrating cranial missile injuries are due to bullets, the mortality is much higher in spite of the fact that there was very rapid evacuation to an excellent neurosurgical unit. The mortality for all of these wounds, minor as well as major, was 56 per cent but the mortality of bullet wounds traversing the brain was nearly 70 per cent for wounds front-to-back and 85 per cent for side-to-side wounds. This is representative of the results in the best of hands for these very severe wounds, and it would be true to say that there are virtually no survivors from a penetrating high velocity bullet wound from a rifle. The only possibility of survival would be in a patient with a tangential wound. Survivors from low velocity, pistol bullet wounds do, however, occur regularly although some survivors are handicapped by hemiparesis; even they do better than the survivors from severe blunt head injury. Epilepsy occurs in 40–50 per cent of patients who survive severe missile wounds of the head.

Early titanium plate cranioplasty has been used with great success in Belfast to replace part of the skull that has been totally destroyed by the missile wound, this gives an excellent cosmetic result and the incidence of complications has been low.

Spinal cord and cauda equina

The spinal cord and the spinal roots of the cauda equina may be injured in the following ways:

1. Directly by penetrating missiles.
2. Cavitational effects of the missile passing close to the spine.
3. Indirectly as a result of fractures and dislocations.

If there is a complete loss of spinal cord function from the time of injury which has not improved after 24 hours the prognosis for eventual recovery is poor and laminectomy is seldom indicated. A neurological defect that is getting progressively worse is an indication for immediate operation.

In the indirect injuries, spontaneous recovery from paraplegia may occur and when this is probable there is usually evidence of this within the first week after injury.

Damage to the spinal roots of the cauda equina usually results from penetrating injuries involving the lumbar and sacral vertebrae. In these cases the prognosis is relatively good, particularly with regard to motor function, but recovery may be delayed for several weeks.

In non-fatal injuries with associated spinal cord damage, later death is most commonly due to urine infections or to sepsis from bed sores. In incomplete lesions spontaneous recovery of cord functions may be seriously interfered with by these complications and their severity depends to a large extent on the treatment given in the first few days. An accurate neurological examination is essential and in particular the upper level of sensory impairment is the best guide to the level of the cord injury. All wounds of the spinal cord should be treated by a neurosurgeon when possible.

When spinal injury results from a penetrating missile, the wound must be thoroughly excised in the fashion already described for soft tissue wounds. Commonly the missile will have damaged chest, neck or abdomen and the management of these wounds will take priority over the spinal wound. At the time of wound excision the spinal cord should not be interfered with. This is because cord damage is almost always due to the shock wave and cavitational effects off the missile, rather than to the physical pressure of a retained fragment. All fragments of missiles and bone are removed and the dura must be closed, the wound should be left open and covered with an absorbant dressing and benzyl penicillin and sulphadiazine should be started as soon as possible after injury. Under ideal circumstances the neurosurgeon will deal with these injuries from the start but if this is not practicable the treatment outlined will ensure that the patient arrives in good condition. At a later stage the neurosurgeon may perform laminectomy for persistent cerebrospinal fluid fistula, progressive spinal compression from haemorrhage, gross deformity of the spine, thecal foreign body in an incomplete spinal lesion or other specific indications.

Dislocations of the cervical spine and flexion fractures may be caused by the tertiary effects of the missile or by the blast wave. If immediate paralysis occurs the prognosis is poor, whereas delayed onset is associated with a better prognosis. Delayed paralysis may be caused by haematoma formation or by gradual displacement of the proximal segment of the spinal column and immediate reduction is indicated.

The early management of patients with open or closed injuries of the spinal cord or cauda equina begins immediately and continues until final rehabilitation. Apart from the wound itself, emphasis is placed on scrupulous attention to nursing care, in order to prevent the occurrence of bed sores, the definitive management of the paralysed bladder, care of the bowel, attention to a high fluid intake and to the nutritional requirements of the patient.

Transportation of the paraplegic patient has to be done with great care, but such movements and indeed their nursing care in general are greatly facilitated by the use of a turning frame such as the Stryker or Martin Baker Povey frame.

References and Further Reading

Byrne, D. P., Crockard, H. A., Gordon, D. S. and Gleadhill, C. A. (1974). Penetrating cranio-cerebral missile injuries in the civil disturbances in Northern Ireland. *British Journal of Surgery*, **61**, 169–76.

Cairns, H. (1947). Neurosurgery in the British Army 1939–1945. *British Journal of Surgery*. War Surgery Supplement, **1**, 9–26.

Crockard, H. A. (1973). The surgery of civil violence – gunshot wounds of the head. In: *Recent Advances of Surgery* ed Taylor, S. Churchill Livingstone, Edinburgh and London, pp 330–4.

Crockard, H. A., Coppel, D. L, and Morrow, W. F. K. (1973). Evaluation of hyperventilation in treatment of head injuries. *British Medical Journal*, **4**, 634–9.

Cushing, H. (1918). A study of a series of wounds of the brain. *British Journal of Surgery*, **5**, 558–604.

Gordon, D. S. (1975). Missile wounds of the head and spine. *British Medical Journal* **1**, 614–16.

Hammon, W. M. (1971). Analysis of 2187 consecutive penetrating wounds of the brain from Vietnam. *Journal of Neurosurgery*, **34**, 127–31.

Small, J. M. and Turner, E. A. (1947). A surgical experience of 1200 cases of penetrating brain wounds in battle in North West Europe 1944–45. *British Journal of Surgery*, War Surgery Supplement, **1**, 62–74.

Small, J. M. and Turner, E. A. and Watt, A. C. (1947). The management of brain wounds in the forward area. *British Journal of Surgery*, War Surgery Supplement **1**, 75–80.

13
Maxillofacial wounds

Maxillofacial wounds from missiles can pose major problems of management. Many of these wounds are horrific to see and have a profound influence on the morale of the patient and those who treat such wounds. Ideally all maxillofacial wounds should have their definitive treatment in the specialized units which are staffed by orodental surgeons, plastic surgeons, ENT surgeons, ophthalmic and neurosurgeons. In such a unit, multiple system wounds of the head and neck can usually be dealt with under the same anaesthetic in a concerted approach by the team of specialists. However, many of these wounds will have to be dealt with by general surgeons, certainly in the first phase of treatment and they must be fully aware of the methods and aims of their specialist colleagues in order to do the correct operation at the time of initial wound surgery.

Most maxillofacial wounds carry the risk of blockage of the airway by accumulated blood clots, by secretions, by loose fragments of teeth or dentures and additional hazards to the airway come from an unstable tongue and from hyoid injuries. The essential first-aid of these wounds is, as always, to maintain the airway by strict attention to clearing the mouth and pharynx, ensuring the tongue is pulled forward and by stopping accessible haemorrhage. It may be necessary to use an oropharyngeal airway, an endotracheal tube or on some occasions a nasotracheal tube in order to maintain an adequate airway. Transport during evacuation for the conscious patient may be with him sitting up with the head held forward so that bleeding and the tongue do not obstruct the airway, or in the prone position with the forehead supported. If the patient is unconscious, then the usual precautions and attention to the airway must be carried out and transport should be in the semiprone position.

Profuse bleeding is common and it may well be necessary to commence resuscitation using intravenous therapy and to stop accessible haemorrhage by packing as an interim measure. Diagnosis includes a careful physical examination paying particular attention to any distortion of the bony landmarks of the face, the level of the eyes, the presence of diplopia or alteration in ocular movements. A specific check should be made to see whether there is any leak of cerebrospinal fluid

146

from the ear or the nose and particular care should be taken over the examination of the mouth and teeth.

Once the airway has been established and haemorrhage controlled, the immediate urgency of the situation in maxillofacial wounds is ended. Their priority for treatment is lowered and although early soft tissue treatment is ideal it is possible that primary treatment can be delayed without adverse effects. This means that such patients can usually await the care of the maxillofacial unit. The principles of management of these wounds are that the damaged tissues should be thoroughly excised, but wounds of the face and neck are one of the few exceptions to the rule for delayed primary closure and may be closed, primarily, with good results. Approach the injury 'inside out and from the bottom of the face upwards' (Small, 1971). The key to restoration of the form and function of the facial skeleton is interdigitation of the teeth in a position of occlusion that is considered acceptable for the patient. Thus alignment of the teeth and alveolar segments is to be accomplished first and the restored segments brought together into occlusion. Finally the remaining facial-skeletal injuries are repaired and the soft tissues closed proceeding outwards from mucosa to the skin. It is important to close the oral mucosa meticulously and to produce a watertight closure over any associated fractures. When there is bone destruction in association with extensive soft tissue damage, it may be necessary to suture buccal mucosa to skin order to cover the fracture site. If the oral cavity has not been sealed by a watertight closure any facture site should be drained to the exterior for a few days. The management of loose bony fragments is similar to that for fractures of bone elsewhere, all tiny fragments are removed but all attached fragments should be cleaned and repositioned. In the face, all fractures should be covered by healthy soft tissue after repositioning them by internal or external fixation methods. Large gaps in the mandible need to be kept in correct alignment and separation using K-wires or similar spacers.

Teeth which are completely loose and fractured teeth with exposed pulp should be removed. Immobilization of the jaw is not only necessary for management of fractures but also facilitates healing of the associated soft tissue wounds. Immobilization is a specialized technique and the hazards have to be weighed in balance with the advantages gained by the procedure. Remember that there is little to be gained by immediate operation on a patient with a good airway. His interests are better served by calm evacuation to a maxillofacial unit for operation after some delay.

References and Further Reading

Converse, J. M. (1974). *Surgical Treatment of Facial Injuries.* Williams and Wilkins, Baltimore.

Fry, W. K. (1953). *Maxillofacial Injuries. History of the Second World War: Surgery.* HMSO, London.

Kelly, J. F. (ed) (1977). *Management of War Injuries of the Jaws and Related Structures.* US Government Printing Office, Washington DC.

Rowe, N. L. and Killey, H. C. (1980). *Fractures of the Facial Skeleton.* 3rd Ed. Williams and Wilkins, Baltimore.

Small, E. W. (1971). Inside out and bottom up. The management of maxillofacial trauma patients. *Military Medicine,* **136,** 553–7.

14
Ear

The ear may be divided into three parts, the external ear, the middle ear and the inner ear. There are four functions related to the ear – the cosmetic appearance, hearing, balance and facial expression mediated through the facial nerve.

Missiles and explosive blast injury can have effects on all four functions of the ear. We must remember that in bomb blast explosions many patients will be deafened and it will, therefore, be difficult to communicate with them.

Cosmetic appearance

Trauma to the external ear is usually quite obvious and unless it is treated correctly may well result in considerable deformity. In simple lacerations the damaged tissues of the auricle should be carefully excised. The laceration should then be closed primarily in layers, being careful to attain good apposition of the cartilage using absorbable suture material like Dexon; the skin and subcutaneous tissues should be closed with fine atraumatic sutures. Lacerations of the external auditory canal should be repaired precisely and it is most important to keep the meatus open afterwards as there is a great tendency for stenosis to occur. When stenosis is a danger a simple obturator, such as a piece of wide bore polythene tubing, can be utilized and this would normally need to be inserted and managed by an ENT surgeon because of the danger of damage to the eardrum.

Hearing

Damage to hearing can be done in three ways. First, the closed or penetrating head injury with or without fracture of the skull. This can result from direct trauma to the head from hand-held weapons, hand-thrown missiles, low and high velocity missiles or from the patient being knocked over by the energy of a missile. Secondly, the temporal bone itself may be actually penetrated by the missiles and thirdly blast trauma to the ear can occur.

Head injury
Head injuries involving the temporal bone may be broadly divided into two types. A longitudinal fracture of the temporal bone may result from a blow on the temple or parietal region and the fracture line involves the squamous temporal bone and runs along the roof of the external auditory meatus, across the roof of the middle ear and anterior to the bony labyrinth usually ending up in the region of the carotid canal. This results in some degree of conductive deafness and usually only a little inner ear deafness. Less commonly, a transverse fracture of the petrous temporal bone occurs. This usually results from a blow on the forehead or in the occipital region and the fracture line runs transversely from the internal auditory meatus into the middle ear bisecting the inner ear and causing complete deafness, and with it severe vertigo. The facial nerve may also be involved in this type of fracture. Usually there is no bleeding from the external auditory meatus although blood may be seen in the middle ear behind an intact eardrum. The deafness is permanent.

Missile injury
Missiles can cause deafness by direct injury to the ear as well as causing indirect injury by virtue of any skull fracture they produce. The direct injury is usually caused by penetration of the temporal bone. These direct injuries are very variable depending upon the size, shape and energy of the missile and on the structures in the ear with which it comes into contact.

Blast injury
There are a number of features of explosive blast that influence damage that is caused to the ear. These are the speed with which the pressure builds up, the maximum peak overpressure and the duration of the positive pressure wave. Blast can damage the hearing in the following three ways:
1. Rupture of the tympanic membrane
2. Dislocation of the ossicles
3. Damage to the inner ear

   Blast damage is much more likely to occur close to the explosion. The ear facing the blast usually suffers greater damage, but there may be occasions when the reflective blast wave from a wall or other solid object may cause damage to the other ear.

Management of hearing damage
Missile injuries may require early exploration, but this is never purely

because of deafness. Life-saving and limb-saving measures must take precedence over the ear problem.

Many of the hearing damaged patients will have bleeding from the ear. In the absence of a recent history of the discharging ear the best course is to do nothing. No attempt should be made to clean up from the ear canal because of the risk of contamination. Sterile cotton wool may be placed at the entrance of the external auditory meatus. If necessary blood can be cleaned out by the ENT surgeon at a later date and the hearing then assessed. If contamination causes middle ear infection, this should be treated by systemic antibiotics.

The majority of cerebrospinal fluid leaks caused by head injuries will close spontaneously. If they fail to stop, exploration of the appropriate area, usually the middle cranial fossa, is necessary to locate and close the hole in the dura.

Inner ear deafness is more difficult to assess because although it is doubtful if anything is effective in the acute phase in restoring hearing, there is certainly nothing that is effective at any later stage. Blast commonly causes severe inner ear deafness which tends to recover rapidly and spontaneously. A few minutes after an explosion, the patient may be unable to hear at all, a few hours later it may have improved although he still may be severely deaf and two days later the hearing may have returned almost to normal. Given the natural history of this response to damage it is virtually impossible to devise any clinical trial of treatment. Unfortunately, full recovery is not always the case and some patients are left with inner ear deafness. In addition, many of these patient's injuries are very extensive and they may have other injuries which prevent the specific treatment of deafness.

Inner ear deafness as the result of blast injuries may be of all degrees of severity. If, when the patient is first seen, the deafness is only mild all treatment may be withheld. If the deafness is moderate a vasodilator such as thymoxamine may be prescribed and if it is severe, a vasodilator, steroids and intravenous low molecular weight Dextran should be given. There is some evidence that these measures are effective and improve the prognosis and provided there are no contraindications, the patient should be given the benefit of early treatment when they have severe inner ear deafness.

Prognosis

Head injuries
With longitudinal fractures of the temporal bone, the middle ear component of deafness often recovers spontaneously and if not, surgical correction is usually possible. The inner ear deafness of the longitudinal

fracture may recover to some extent, but that resulting from the transverse fracture is usually total and permanent.

Missiles
In missile injuries, the prognosis depends upon the severity of the damage to the middle and inner ear.

Blast
Kerr and Byrne (1975) analysed in considerable detail all the casualties from the 5 lb bomb in the Abercorn Restaurant in Belfast. There were 60 perforated eardrums from this explosion. The majority of these healed spontaneously, 11 did not and seven had been operated on with success. Most of the people in the explosion suffered immediate inner ear deafness, but the majority made a good recovery. About one-third had some degree of permanent inner ear deafness, with high frequency sensineural loss of hearing greater than 30 dB for 4000 and 8000 Hz in both ears. About 5 per cent of the total injured had bilateral persistant deafness of at least moderate severity, and these could be said to have suffered severe inner ear damage.

Balance

There are three main causes of dizziness following missile blast injuries involving the ear or the head. They are:
1. Destruction of the vestibular labyrinth
2. Postconcussional vertigo
3. Benign positional vertigo

Destruction of the vestibular labyrinth
The most dramatic dizziness occurs after complete destruction of the vestibular apparatus. The clinical picture is that of vomiting, associated with severe dizziness even when still and increasing with the slightest movement of the head. Examination will show horizontal nystagmus. This injury usually occurs after penetrating missile injuries or transverse fractures of the temporal bone. At the time of admission, the presence or absence of nystagmus and its direction should be recorded. The patient should also be kept still because head movement tends to precipitate vomiting and labyrinth sedative drugs such as Cyclizine are of considerable help. The dizziness will improve gradually, but it is usually some days before he is able to walk unaided.

Postconcussional vertigo
This usually takes the form of postural dizziness on rising from the sitting position and this gradually improves without treatment.

Benign positional vertigo

In this condition the patient suffers from severe but short lived rotatory vertigo which is precipitated by certain head positions. It is due to the deposition of calcium on the cupula of one of the posterior semicircular canals. The condition is readily diagnosed by the demonstration of rotatory nystagmus in the positional test. It is a self-limiting condition which, in the majority of cases, settles spontaneously within one to two years. The condition may be readily confused with postconcussional vertigo.

The facial nerve

The facial nerve lies in a narrow bony canal and runs a tortuous course through the temporal bone. Facial nerve paralysis may be immediate or delayed. Immediate facial paralysis indicates that there has been direct damage to the nerve at the time of the injury, and delayed paralysis indicates secondary oedema of the nerve, probably as the result of alteration of its vascular supply. It is vitally important to establish, on admission of the patient, that facial nerve function is normal or otherwise.

Immediate damage to the facial nerve in association with a fracture of the skull, is likely to be due to tearing of the nerve or to impaction of bone into the nerve. Good recovery of nerve function cannot occur without operation and exploration should, therefore, be carried out as soon as possible after the injury.

When facial paralysis occurs after a delay, the prognosis is quite different from that of immediate paralysis. If the delayed paralysis does not progress further and remains incomplete, then there should usually be full recovery. If the paralysis does become complete there is still good chances of recovery, but it has been shown that the use of steroids improves the prognosis. Therefore, provided there are no contraindications, delayed facial paralysis should be treated with ACTH in a dose of 80 units a day for five days with decreasing doses over the next five days.

References and Further Reading

Kerr, A. G. and Byrne, J. E. T. (1975). Blast injuries of the ear. *British Medical Journal*, **1,** 559–61.

Kerr, A. G. and Byrne, J. E. T. (1975). Concussive effects of bomb blast on the ear. *Proceedings of the Royal Society of Medicine*, **67,** 131–43.

Smyth, G. D. L. and Stewart, T. J. (1973). The surgery of civil violence – injuries to the ear. In *Recent Advances in Surgery*, ed. Taylor, S. Churchill Livingstone, Edinburgh and London, pp. 337–8.

15
Eye

The eye may be damaged by penetrating fragments from primary or secondary missiles, by the explosive blast pressure wave and by severe blunt trauma. All ocular injuries are potentially serious and the distinction between minor and major is not always easy to make, for even the most trivial looking injury may be very serious. Even serious injuries, if properly managed, may result in some salvage of vision. All these wounds are dangerous to deal with unless a surgeon is experienced in the special skills and techniques of ophthalmic surgery and has the special instruments required for their performance. The first chance of repair of an ocular injury is usually the last and disaster from improper treatment leaves no room for later remedies by the most skilled surgeon. Although the eyes are injured in up to 10 per cent of all non-fatal casualties in war, most wounds of the eye from missiles and bomb blast injury do not occur in isolation and the patient's injuries must be evaluated as a whole. Nevertheless, any eye injury must be seen by the opthalmologist as soon as it is feasible so that he can assess the importance of the eye injury in terms of the whole person and carry out emergency treatment until such time as he can be given access to the patient's eyes.

The first-aid treatment for all ocular wounds is to apply a sterile pad to the affected eye. Great care should be taken that no pressure is applied to the damaged eye whilst applying this pad.

Emergency treatment by the first surgeon to see the patient is to assess the degree of ocular damage so that he may inform the ophthalmologist of the details. The type of wounding agent and the circumstances in which the injury was acquired should be recorded and then each eye should be examined separately, taking particular care that at this stage no pressure at all is applied to the globe. The eye should be thoroughly irrigated with copious amounts of plain sterile water or normal saline solution and under local anaesthetic if necessary. Inspection and testing visual acuity should be done with the lids retracted. Visual acuity should be recorded as follows:
1. No perception of light
2. Perception of light

3. Perception of motion in the field of view
4. Counts fingers
5. Reads print

The light used for testing should be a bright light with the other eye completely shielded. Inspection of the eye may reveal irregularity of the pupil, hyphaema or even collapse of the anterior chamber, lacerations of the eyelids, cornea or sclera, prolapse of the iris, foreign bodies within the eye or the orbit or disruption of the globe may be present. Finally the ocular movements should be tested and recorded.

In the temporary absence of an opthalmologist, treatment must be limited to measures which reduce the risk of infection within the eye. Systemic antibiotics will have been started and tetanus toxoid booster given. The lids and conjunctivae should be thoroughly and freely irrigated and then a generous application of antibiotic solution such as chloramphenicol, gentamycin or neomycin-polymyxin together with 1 per cent atropine. The eye should then be covered with a sterile pad. No ocular surgery should be performed, and in particular no attempt should be made to remove any penetrating or protruding foreign bodies or to repair any corneoscleral lacerations. The patient and the staff must be instructed not to squeeze the eyes or eyelids, under any circumstances, to any degree. Delay is acceptable to the ophthalmologist in order that he be the first to commence primary surgical treatment for all ocular injuries.

References and Further Reading

Deroe, A. G. (1974). Penetrating wounds of the anterior segment. *International Ophthalmological Clinics*, **14,** 99–110.
Maltzman, B. H. (1975). Prognosis and treatment of perforating ocular injuries. *Surgical Forum* **25,** 503–5.
Maguire, C. J. F. and Johnston, S. S. (1973). The surgery of civil violence – ocular injuries, in *Recent Advances in Surgery*, Taylor, S. Churchill Livingstone, Edinburgh and London, pp. 334–7.
Duke-Elder, S. (ed) (1972). *System of Ophthalmology*, Vol. XIV Part 1, Mechanical Injuries. Henry Kimpton, London.
Bailey, Hamilton, (ed) (1942). Wounds of the eye and orbit, in *Surgery of Modern Warfare*, 2nd ed, E & S Livingstone, Edinburgh, pp. 821–65.

16

Genito-urinary tract

About 4–5 per cent of all missile wounds involve the genito-urinary tract. Wounds of the external genitalia may be obvious but most urinary tract injuries will be hidden and such a wound must be suspected in all patients with penetrating injuries of the abdomen, pelvis, loins and buttocks.

The general principle of management of all these injuries is to examine the urine, if necessary passing a catheter. Then:

1. Control haemorrhage
2. Conserve all viable tissue during missile wound excision
3. Divert the urinary stream above the site of injury
4. Drain the sites of urine extravasation
5. Prompt primary repair of wounds of the ureter, urethra or bladder.

Wounds of the kidney

These may be penetrating injuries from bullets or fragments or they may be closed injuries caused by direct trauma from secondary missiles, vehicle accidents or explosive blast injuries. Renal tissue withstands damage quite well and the surgeon should be conservative in his management. The patient must be completely examined so that all his injuries may be evaluated and the priorities established for their treatment. The urine should be examined and plain abdominal radiographs together with intravenous or retrograde urography films, if available, studied. This is important in order to check on the presence and the function of the opposite kidney before operation.

Operative treatment consists of wound excision and removal of dead renal tissue. The surgical approach is usually abdominal in penetrating wounds as it is essential to assess damage to other structures within the abdomen. It is important that the vascular pedicle should be exposed and controlled before opening the perirenal tissues which, despite penetration and breach of the fascial layers may still be localizing the bleeding to some extent within the perirenal fascia.

Nephrectomy is warranted only when the kidney is irretrievably damaged; it is the injury to the vascular supply which will usually determine the operation. In moderately severe injuries, excision of the damaged renal tissue, removal of foreign bodies together with suture of renal and pelvic tears will be necessary. Partial nephrectomy is only rarely required. Nephrectomy may, on occasions, be indicated and in all cases adequate perinephric drainage is mandatory.

Wounds of the ureter

Wounds of the ureter seldom occur in isolation. The wounds usually involve complete transection but occasionally a perforating or lacerating wound may occur. The injury is commonly missed and the possibility must be constantly borne in mind whenever there is penetrating injury associated with a retroperitoneal haematoma or with injuries to the fixed portions of the colon, duodenum and spleen. Sometimes a wound of the ureter is not recognized until urine drains from the external wound or into the peritoneal cavity.

It is important that wounds of the ureter are repaired promptly. Transection of the ureter requires anastomosis with interrupted fine, absorbable sutures over a ureteral catheter, running from renal pelvis to the bladder, which serves as a splint; it is important not to include the mucosa of the ureter in the sutures. The urinary stream must be diverted above the site of injury by ureterostomy using a ureteral catheter or T-tube in order to protect the anastomosis or repair. A minor injury of the ureter can be treated by splinting with a ureteral catheter alone. Injuries of the ureter close to the bladder can be treated by simple reimplantation of the lower end into the bladder, or by a Boari flap.

When immediate repair of the ureter is not feasible, nephrostomy or ureterostomy must be done in order to preserve renal function until time permits a repair. Adequate drainage at the site of the injury to the ureter is always required.

Wounds of the bladder

The full bladder is much more liable to penetrating injuries than is the empty bladder. Bladder injuries are commonly associated with injuries to the pelvic bones, the large bowel and the female internal genitalia.

The diagnosis of injuries to the bladder depends on clinical findings and cystography.

Wounds of the bladder are divided into intraperitoneal and extraperitoneal. The latter also including rupture of the membranous urethra with traumatic avulsion of the triangular ligament; this allows the bladder to float up into the false pelvis.

Management includes examining the urine and performing a simple urethrogram and cystogram. The abdomen is then opened and the bladder examined for the source of leakage of urine and of bleeding. Any laceration is closed using interrupted absorbable sutures in two layers, one taking muscle but not mucosa and the other taking visceral peritoneum. Associated wounds must be dealt with, in particular rectal or sigmoid colon injuries must be repaired and a proximal defunctioning colostomy fashioned. The abdominal incision is then closed, the bladder opened extraperitonealy and a suprapubic cystostomy tube inserted; the prevesical space must always be drained. When intraperitoneal exploration does not reveal the bladder damage, the prevesical space must be opened and the bladder examined to find the laceration. This is then sutured using the technique already described. Suprapubic cystostomy and prevesical drainage are established and if closure is difficult the wound of the bladder may be left open with the suprapubic drain sutured in place. If the bladder neck has been torn away from the triangular ligament, bleeding must be controlled and any bladder injury repaired. A Foley catheter is then passed and manoeuvred into the bladder, it is then inflated and the bladder pulled down to the triangular ligament by light traction, which would need to be maintained for two to three weeks. If the entry wound is through the perineum, the wounds are excised, the bladder closed and suprapubic cystostomy and prevesical drainage performed. Any associated injuries of the prostate, seminal vesicles or female pelvic organs must be dealt with at the same operation.

Wounds of the urethra

The general principles of management include excision of the missile wound, diversion of the urine by suprapubic cystostomy, repair of the urethral injury, either primarily or delayed and adequate wound drainage. In most cases the most practicable treatment is excision of the wound, suprapubic cystostomy and evacuation to a Urology Unit.

The urethra is divided into two parts by the urogenital diaphragm and wounds are usually classified according to whether the anterior or posterior urethra is involved.

Anterior urethra

Penetrating wounds may involve the pendulous or the fixed portions of the urethra. Those of the pendulous portion are treated by wound excision, by repair if the urethral damage is small and by marsupialization if the damage is more extensive. If the urethra is transected fairly cleanly, it should be mobilized carefully and repaired, making sure that there is no tension on the suture line and that there is no constriction of the anastomosis. Wounds of the fixed portion of the anterior urethra should be excised and repaired over a catheter, bringing it out through the perineum if the damage is extensive. In all cases suprapubic cystostomy and wound drainage are provided.

Posterior urethra

Penetrating wounds may divide the posterior urethra cleanly but in most cases the injuries are caused by trauma to the pelvis which causes avulsion of the bladder and prostate from the membraneous urethra. The retropubic space and the bladder must be opened, a Foley catheter manoeuvred through the urethra into the bladder and the balloon inflated. Traction should then pull the bladder and prostate down thus bringing the torn ends of the urethra together. At operation it is advisable to anchor the prostate in place with stout absorbable sutures to the pelvic fascia or through the perineum (Turner-Warwick, 1973) in order to hold the ends of the urethra in apposition and to take the strain off the catheter balloon. Suprapubic cystostomy and drainage of the retropubic space are required and a long suture tied to the tip of the Foley catheter may be brought out through the cystostomy tube in order to facilitate replacement of the catheter if it becomes necessary.

Wounds of the external genitalia

The management of wounds of the penis, scrotum, testes and the spermatic cord consists of control of haemorrhage, conservative wound excision and reconstruction.

When there has been extensive loss of skin, the penis may be placed in a scrotal tunnel until later plastic surgery repair is possible.

In testicular injuries all tissues should be conserved as far as possible and if there is extensive skin loss the testicle may be placed in a protective subcutaneous pocket in the thigh. The surgeon should be as conservative as possible with the skin of the scrotum and penis in order to facilitate later repair.

References and Further Reading

Clarke, B.G. and Leadbetter, W.F. (1952). Management of wounds and injuries of the genito-urinary tract. A review of reported experience in World War II. *Journal of Urology*, **67**, 719–39.

Culp, O.S. (1947). War wounds of the genito-urinary tract. *Journal of Urology*, **57**, 1117–28.

Mitchell, J.P. (1968). Injuries to the urethra. *British Journal of Urology*, **40**, 649–70.

Pontes, J.E. (1977). Urologic injuries. *Surgical Clinics of North America*, **57** (1), 77–96.

Poole-Wilson, D.S. (1949). Missile injuries of the urethra. *British Journal of Surgery*, **36**, 364–76.

Poole-Wilson, D.S. (1952). A survey of patients treated at the genito-urinary centre in the CMF. *British Journal of Surgery*. War Surgery Supplement, **3**, 471–7.

Rohner, T.J. and Blanchard, T.W. (1970). Management of urethral injuries in war casualties. *Military Medicine*, **135**, 748–51.

Salvatierra, O, Rigdon, W.O., Norris, D.M. and Brady, T.W. (1969). Vietnam experience with 252 urological war injuries. *Journal of Urology*, **101**, 615–20.

Selikowitz, S.M. (1977). Penetrating high velocity genito-urinary injuries. *Urology*, **9**, Part I, 371–76; Part II, 493–9.

Stutzman, R.E. (1977). Ballistics and the management of urethral injuries from high velocity missiles. *Journal of Urology*, **118**, 947–49.

Turner-Warwick, R.T. (1973). Observations on the treatment of traumatic urethral injuries and the value of the fenestrated urethral catheter. *British Journal of Surgery*, **60**, 775–81.

Van Buskirk, K.E. and Kimbrough, J.C. (1954). Urological surgery in combat. *Journal of Urology*, **71**, 639–46.

Williams, J.P. (1976). Injuries to the urinary tract. in: *Recent Advances in Surgery*, ed. Hendry, W.F. Churchill Livingstone, Edinburgh and London pp. 113–24.

17
Gas gangrene

Many of the great men of medicine have been interested in gas gangrene as a complication of wounds because of its spectacular nature, fulminating course, profound toxaemia, mutilating effects and high mortality. Hippocrates described vividly a fulminating infection of the leg which appears to have been gas gangrene and Celsus also seemed to have recognized its occurrence. For some strange reason it was not separately described by many of the military surgeons during the wars of the Middle Ages although they must have observed very many wounds. I think probably they just described it as a rapidly advancing gangrene causing death and because they were so used to it they did not think it worth observing closely. In the eighteenth century there were a number of very accurate descriptions, probably the first being Peyronnie who described the 'subcutaneous emphysema, the erysipelatous colour of the skin and the rapidity of death'. Early in the nineteenth century Baron Jean Larrey described the rapid progress of gangrene which spread from the injured limb in a few hours and often caused death in less than ten hours. To prevent this well recognized complication of wounds, which he called 'traumatic gangrene', he advocated early amputation of badly damaged extremities. Billroth anticipated later discoveries by believing that 'the decomposition of mortified elements caused possibly by the action of some ferment, was the cause of this catastrophic condition'. Maisonneuve in 1853 named it 'gangrene foudroyante' and it was about this time that the disease acquired its name as a clinical entity. The condition was widely reported in the Crimean War and in the Franco-Prussian war whereas there does not appear to be any record of it during the American Civil War.

Shortly after this period the bacterial cause of the disease was established and the more important causal bacteria were identified by various workers. Louis Pasteur discovered the *Vibrion septique*, Novy the *Clostridium oedematiens* and Welch the *Clostridium welchii*.

Clostridium welchii is also known as *C. perfringens*, and *C. oedematiens* is also known as *C. novyi*. For personal preference and dating to the time of my early experimental work in the prophylaxis of gas gangrene in animals, I will refer to the main organisms as *C. welchii*, *C. oedematiens* and *C. septicum*.

There were very large numbers of cases of gas gangrene during World War I and according to Zeissler at least 100 000 German soldiers died of this complication. Certainly it was an extremely common condition and has been well described in the writings of that period, with an incidence in many areas of about 10 per cent. Throughout World War II in Europe, Africa and the Far East the incidence varied between 0.3 and 1.5 per cent.

Certain types of penetrating wounds from missiles have produced conditions in which gas gangrene is particularly likely to develop. It is most common in wounds in which there is extensive damage to muscles, particularly those involving buttocks and lower limbs and to a lesser degree in other parts of the body where there are major muscle masses. Ninety per cent of cases involve the extremities with 70 per cent in the buttock, thigh or leg. All high velocity wounds are grossly contaminated and clostridia from the patients own skin will be drawn into the depths of the wound. However, when the wound is grossly contaminated with soil and dirt and with fragments of clothing then the possibility of gross clostridial contamination is obviously much higher. When there has been damage to the main blood supply of the affected part and particularly where operation has been, for various reasons, delayed by difficulties in evacuation or owing to the needs of resuscitation then all these conditions are compounded so that with such a wound there is a high risk indeed of developing gas gangrene.

Gas gangrene is a rapidly spreading oedematous myonecrosis occurring characteristically in association with severe wounds of extensive muscle masses that have been contaminated with pathogenic spore-bearing anaerobes particularly *Clostridium welchii*. Almost every case presents a mixed bacterial flora and it is unusual to have a single organism responsible for the infection. The main organisms are *C. welchii* and *C. oedematiens*, *C. septicum*, *C. histolyticum* and *C. sporogenes*. There are a number of other clostridia which can be identified but are of less importance. The different strains have varied symbiotic and synergistic relationships which are still not fully understood. The bacteria producing the initial infection in gas gangrene are only slightly proteolytic and much of the tissue destruction and digestion that follows the infection is thought to be due to proteolytic commensals, the most frequent and active of these being *C. sporogenes*.

C. welchii is extremely widely distributed in nature, it can be isolated from the faeces in almost every case and is widely distributed in the dirt of buildings and streets and in the soil. The features of the disease are due, first to a local action of the organisms on the sugar of the muscle, producing acid and gas (the saccharolytic group) and on muscle protein causing digestion (the proteolytic group); second, to the production by the organisms of soluble, very potent toxins which diffuse into the tissues causing further tissue destruction and a profound toxaemia. The breakdown products of the muscle from the effects of the toxin are profoundly toxic in their own right and it is this combination of breakdown products and specific toxins that cause the relentless and profound toxaemia which untreated will inevitably lead to death.

In large muscle wounds there will always be found areas of ischaemia; the consequent reduction in pH allows the clostridia to multiply and the toxins to be produced. It is not always necessary for the trauma to be very severe; provided the wound is deep, contains necrotic tissue and is shut off from the surface it is always possible for an anaerobic infection to become established and there are records of many hundreds of cases of gas gangrene following hypodermic injections, particularly the injection of adrenalin. For exactly similar reasons, the presence of foreign bodies in the wound such as clothing, soil, metal or wood or the prolonged application of a tourniquet or tight plaster will increase the liability of the injured person to the disease, for such conditions will produce local ischaemia and anoxia in the wound. The influence of delay in treatment is even more obvious and is the main reason why gas gangrene is so much more common during conditions of war.

The incubation period of gas gangrene is usually short almost always less than three days and in the majority of cases less than 24 hours. It has occasionally occurred at intervals up to six weeks and incubation periods of less than one hour are on record. It is also worth noting that clostridial spores may remain dormant in scar tissue for considerable periods and then give rise to gas gangrene years after the original injury as a result of quite minor trauma which may not even involve a penetrating injury. Typically gas gangrene manifests itself with the sudden appearance of pain in the region of the wound. The sudden onset of pain, sometimes so sudden as to suggest a vascular catastrophe, should always make one consider the possibility of gas gangrene in a wounded man.

Soon after the patient complains of pain, local swelling and oedema and a thin often haemorrhagic exudate can be observed. There is a marked rise in the pulse rate but as a rule only a slight elevation of the temperature, rarely to more than 38°C (100° F); indeed in some cases it is sub-normal. The most striking feature is a rapid change for the worse in a wounded man who, until then, had been progressing satisfactorily; in the course of a few hours he becomes anxious, frightened or euphoric, his face is pale or livid, often with marked circumoral pallor. A rising pulse in a man wounded by a high velocity missile, who has recovered from shock and is not suffering from continued haemorrhage is highly suggestive of the development of gas gangrene. The blood pressure is usually low, vomiting may be a feature in severe cases and there is practically no response to blood transfusion. Unless immediate surgical measures are undertaken the case goes on to a condition of utter prostration, rapidly fatal.

It should be emphasized that gas is not obvious at the earlier stages and may well be completely absent. At most, a certain frothiness of the exudate may be noted, for the oedematous area is too tender to permit deep palpation. The skin is tense, white, often marbled with blue, and rather colder than normal. Rarely, slight bronzing may be seen around the taut edges of the wound, particularly if haemolytic streptococci are present. The pathological process advances rapidly. The swelling, oedema and toxaemia increase, the serous discharge becomes more and more profuse and in most cases a peculiar, sweetish smell will be sensed. This smell is very variable and although regarded by many experienced observers who have seen many cases in war-time, as highly suggestive of gas gangrene it is not pathognomonic. Undoubtedly many cases occur in which the smell is either absent or masked by the general odour of putrefaction. In addition to the state of shock so characteristic of gas gangrene toxaemia, usually certain peculiar mental changes, consisting of great intellectual clarity, complete appreciation of the gravity of the circumstances, and a most profound and distressing terror of impending death. This is particularly true with *C. welchii* infections which are by far the most common and persist almost to the end. In untreated cases the local bronzing of the skin becomes more diffuse; greenish yellow areas occur in which blebs may form; these may become filled with dark red fluid and patches of cutaneous gangrene may occur. Gas is usually produced at this stage and is partly responsible for the swelling of the affected part. It is produced in and between the muscle fibres and eventually escapes into the subcutaneous tissues under pressure through holes in the fascia from where it spreads rapidly beyond the confines of the infected area. The skin may, however, appear normal even when lying over massive gangrene and neither the cutaneous changes nor any clinically demonstrable gas are as extensive as the involvement of the underlying muscle.

The infection spreads up and down the muscle from the site of the wound and has little tendency to spread to other healthy muscles. Even in well established gas gangrene the blood stream is rarely invaded by clostridia until immediately before death. The muscle changes are usually only seen at operation; in the earlier stage they consist of little more than swelling and pallor, later the colour alters to a lustreless pinkish-grey, then to a brick red, then to a very typical slate blue colour and finally to a dark green purple.

In *C. oedematiens* infections, gas may well be entirely absent; there is a profuse golden yellow discharge from the wound and the muscles become almost slimy and firm to the touch. Later on they become dark red, purple and soft. The toxaemia is quite out of proportion to any obvious local lesion. The mental changes are usually slight and the patient is commonly apathetic.

In *C. septicum* infections the course is even more acute than the other two described. The onset is abrupt, with severe pain in the affected part, great swelling occurs and an erythematous flush develops around the wound which exudes large quantities of bright red haemorrhagic fluid. Gas is usually a prominent feature even early in the disease. The affected muscles are quite typical: they are a startling red colour, mottled and commonly barred with purple. The toxaemia is great and elevation of the temperature to 39°C (102° F) or more is common and delirium is usual.

The common mixed infections tend to give symptoms and signs which are a combination of those described for the specific organisms. Other clostridia are usually involved in most of the infections and many of them are of minor importance. However, each of the separate types produces its own specific toxins and, to some extent, each may be said to give rise to a slightly different disease. A further complication is the occurrence of more than one species of toxigenic clostridium in the same case.

All the clostridia can be divided into a number of different groups, each group of which tends to produce a particular disease either in man or in animals. Each clostridia within a group produces a combination of many toxins, two or three of which are the most important associated with a particular disease; e.g. in *C. welchii* type A the main toxins produced are the α, θ and κ types. The α toxin, which is a lecithinase, is haemolytic, dermonecrotizing and lethal and is certainly the most important constituent of type A toxic filtrates. The other clostridia have similar groupings of potent toxins that have been isolated. It must be remembered, however, that the toxins are not the direct cause of death ing gas gangrene; rather it is the product of their action on dead muscle which produces breakdown products which are so toxic. So although antitoxins will stop the activity of the toxins and thus disarm the clostridia producing them, it must always be supplemented by excision of the dead muscle if the patient is to survive.

Active immunization against the main clostridial toxins is possible; it has been common practice in animals against specific diseases for many years. Experimentally it is possible to protect large animals against a high velocity missile wound of muscle deliberately contaminated with clostridial spores, which in unprotected controls results in rapid death from gas gangrene (Boyd *et al.*, 1972 a, b). Human volunteers obtain adequate blood levels of antibodies following active immunization; in theory they could be protected against developing gas gangrene from such a wound (Adams, 1947; Tytell *et al.*, 1947).

Passive immunization has been much more widely used. In animals effective protection from gas gangrene has been obtained in experimental work for over fifty years. Effective protection in large sheep was shown in 1968 (Owen-Smith) in high velocity bullet wounds contaminated with *C. oedematiens*. With no other treatment the animals survived, whereas the controls died rapidly of gas gangrene. Treatment could be delayed for up to nine hours with no ill effect but further delay was fatal. The animals developed an abscess in the muscle, which caused minimal disability, but from which *C. oedematiens* could be seen on direct gram stain and of course could be cultured (Boyd, *et al.*, 1972 a, b).

Much ignorance and prejudice against clostridial antitoxins still exists. In war wounds with massive tissue destruction in large muscle masses, the risk of gas gangrene is relatively high. The contamination is greater; there is inevitable delay to surgery and the muscle damage is commonly greater than in civil practice. Those with very wide experience of the use of clostridial antitoxins in high risk cases in World War II had no doubts whatsoever of the prophylactic value, but emphasized that it must be combined with excision of the dead and contaminated muscle and with the use of penicillin to kill the bacteria (MacLennan and Macfarlane, 1944).

Those with little or no experience of its use denigrate its value and comments that it is useless and dangerous have been copied from one textbook to another without weighing the evidence and often in ignorance of work done in this particular field. It has been effective in many hundreds of human cases, battle casualties and others; the experimental work is unequivocal and I firmly believe that antiserum should be a part of the armamentarium against gas gangrene. I fully accept that it plays a subsidiary role because early and thorough surgery, early use of penicillin and the use of hyperbaric oxygen should obviate the need for antiserum but we must remember that patients still die from gas gangrene even in the most developed countries and in modern hospitals using modern techniques and the latest antibiotics!

The antiserum vial normally contains 10 000 iu of *C. welchii* and *C. oedematiens* and 5000 iu of *C. septicum* antitoxins; the dose is normally one vial intramuscularly or by slow intravenous injection and can be repeated 12-hourly if necessary. Provided surgery can be performed to remove the contaminated tissues there should be little need for any further doses.

By far the most important technique in the prophylaxis of gas gangrene in missile wounds is early and adequate surgery. Thorough excision of the dead tissues, actively contaminated by the cavitation process of the missile, together with the early use of penicillin, will virtually eliminate gas gangrene. When there is delay to surgery, such as in a full scale war situation or in a civilian disaster with mass casualties overwhelming the medical service, then gas gangrene will rear its ugly head. We must remember that it is the driving force behind the necessity for establishing the principles of surgery for high velocity missile wounds.

Antibiotics like penicillin, tetracycline and erythromycin are effective against *Clostridia* organisms but they can only reach tissues with an active blood supply and good tissue perfusion. Dead muscle allows diffusion only and antibiotic concentrations in the depths of the wound are very low and ineffective. All patients with high velocity missile wounds should receive benzyl penicillin in a dose of 1 megaunit repeated 6-hourly for five days. If the patient is sensitive to penicillin then they should receive tetracycline, although some clostridia may rarely be resistant to this, or erythromycin.

Finally we must remember that in missile wounds clostridial contamination ranges from 30 per cent upwards. Growing clostridia on culture from these wounds is normal; only a tiny proportion actually go on to develop infection and clostridial cellulitis.

Anaerobic cellulitis was well described by Qvist (1941) as a heavy clostridial infection involving necrotic tissue which has already been killed, not by bacterial action, but by ischaemia or direct trauma. Intact, healthy muscle is not invaded. In a typical case there is a history of injury several days previously, with the gradual appearance of a foul wound exuding an evil smelling, brownish, seropurulent discharge and with obvious gas bubbling through the fluid and present in the tissues. The gas is never found intramuscularly; it is far more obvious than in gas gangrene; there is little oedema and no discolouration of the skin. For treatment all that is required is the relief of tension, the removal of necrotic tissue leaving the wound open for delayed closure and the use of antibiotics. One must be as wary of being too ruthless with clostridial cellulitis as one is of not being ruthless enough in gas gangrene.

Even fewer develop gas gangrene which, it is emphasized again, is a clinical diagnosis not a bacteriological one, and with a proper understanding of its aetiology hopefully it can be virtually eliminated in high velocity wounds.

References and Further Reading

Adams, M.H. (1947). Antigenicity of gas gangrene toxoids in guinea-pigs, mice and human beings. *Journal of Immunology*, **56**, 323–35.

168   *Gas gangrene*

Boyd, N.A., Walker, P.D. and Thomson, R.O. (1972a). The prevention of experimental *C. novyi* gas gangrene in high velocity missile wounds by passive immunisation. *Journal of Medical Microbiology*, **5**, 459–65.

Boyd, N.A., Walker, P.D. and Thomson, R.O. (1972b). The prevention of experimental *C. novyi* and *C. perfringens* gas gangrene in high velocity missile wounds by active immunisation. *Journal of Medical Microbiology*, **5**, 467–72.

Evans, D.G. (1945). Treatment with antitoxin of experimental gas gangrene produced in guinea-pigs. *British Journal of Experimental Pathology*, **26**, 104–11.

Garrod, L.P. (1958). The chemoprophylaxis of gas gangrene. *Journal of the Royal Army Medical Corps*, **104**, 208–15.

Macfarlane, M.G. (1945). Case fatality rates of gas gangrene in relation to treatment. *British Medical Journal*, **1**, 803–6.

MacLennan, J.D. (1943). Anaerobic infections of war wounds in the Middle East. *Lancet*, **2**, 63–6, 94–9, 123–6.

MacLennan, J.D. (1962). The histotoxic Clostridial infections of man. *Bacteriological Reviews*, **26** (2), 177–276.

MacLennan, J.D. and Macfarlane, M.G. (1944). The treatment of gas gangrene. *British Medical Journal*, **2**, 683–5.

Oakley, C.L. (1954). Gas gangrene. *British Medical Bulletin*, **10**, 52–8.

Owen-Smith, M.S. (1968). Antibiotics and antitoxin therapy in the prophylaxis of experimental gas gangrene. *British Journal of Surgery*, **55**, 43–5.

Owen-Smith, M.S. (1971). *The Successful Prophylaxis of Gas Gangrene*. MS Thesis, University of London.

Owen-Smith, M.S. and Matheson, J.M. (1968). Successful prophylaxis of gas gangrene in the high velocity missile wound in sheep. *British Journal of Surgery*, **55**, 36–9.

Qvist, G. (1941). Anaerobic cellulitis and gas gangrene. *British Medical Journal*, **2**, 217–21.

Robb-Smith, A.H.T. (1945). Tissue changes induced by *C. welchii* type A filtrates. *Lancet*, **2**, 362–8.

Thoresby, F.P. and Watts, J.C. (1967). Gas gangrene of the high velocity missile wound. *British Journal of Surgery*, **54**, 25–9.

Tytell, A.A., Logan, M.A., Tytell, A.G. and Tepper, J (1947). Immunisation of humans and animals with gas gangrene toxoids. *Journal of Immunology*, **55**, 233–44.

18
Shot-gun wounds

Shot-guns are long barrelled, smooth-bore guns and create a rather different type of wound from those of the rifled weapons like pistols and rifles. The cartridge consists of a pressed paper or plastic casing, seated in a metal detonator cap. The propellant powder is separated from the shot by wadding made of paper, felt, plastic or cork. The shot is usually lead spheres and are described by the number of them that there are to the ounce. The bore or gauge of the shot-gun refers to the number of spherical lead balls of the correct bore that weigh one pound. The shot and the wadding are projected from the barrel on firing the gun in the shape of a rapidly expanding core and is designed so as to hit small birds or game with at least one lead shot. The effective range is about 20–50 m because the spherical lead shot are not streamlined like a bullet and rapidly slow up due to the resistance of air. The shot-gun is lethal at short ranges of 10–15 m when the whole mass of the shot produces an extensive wound. At these ranges each shot acts as a high velocity missile and the total effect is the sum of the damage from many missiles.

Shot-gun wounds may be classified into three types based on the range, the pattern of shot distribution and the depth of penetration. Type 1 injuries are those wounds in which only the subcutaneous tissue and deep fascia are penetrated and this usually occurs at extended ranges. Type 2 wounds are inflicted at close range and the structures beneath the deep fascia are perforated. Type 3 occur at point blank range of less than 5 m and produce immense tissue destruction, they usually take the form of a large hole in the tissue with a small surrounding halo of pellet holes.

Management

Type 1 wounds are best treated by cleansing thoroughly and applying a sterile dressing. The pellets may be removed if they present, as they are not very deeply embedded. Type 2 wounds, that have penetrated the deep fascia, may produce a significant injury although the wound may appear innocent. All these wounds should be explored in the same way as for other penetrating bullet wounds in similar areas as has already been described. Type 3 injuries are commonly associated with massive tissue destruction, multiple organ injury and major surface defects. It is this latter problem that creates the main distinction between the management of shot-gun wounds and those from rifle bullets.

Type 3 wounds of the extremity produce massive muscle injury, comminuted fractures and commonly damage large segments of artery and vein. The most important decision to be made is whether the limb is salvageable or whether amputation is required. The principles of treatment are similar to those for a severe high velocity bullet wound, i.e. thorough excision of the dead tissues, haemostasis, fasciotomy, vein graft to damaged arteries and veins and skeletal fixation by traction or external fixation devices.

Abdominal injuries from shot-guns quite commonly cause a large full thickness abdominal wall defect. The prognosis of the patient depends upon the intra-abdominal injuries but presuming that these can be repaired the main factor that determines morbidity and mortality is the management of the full thickness of the abdominal wall defect. The immediate use of prosthetic materials has commonly lead to severe wound sepsis and a practical alternative is based on the technique utilizing an abdominal pack placed over a sheet of porous material like rayon cloth which lies directly on the viscera. The pack is held in place by retention sutures placed well beyond the wound margin and these serve to maintain the viscera within the peritoneal cavity. The abdominal wall pack may be changed every two to three days and the underlying rayon cloth may be removed after about ten days by which time a layer of granulation tissue has formed over the exposed viscera. This granulation tissue should be encouraged by repeated application of porcine skin graft until the wound is ready for autografting. Six months later the abdominal wall can be reconstructed by excising the skin graft and closing the defect by rotation of flaps or the use of prosthetic material.

Thoracic wall defects from massive shot-gun wounds rarely result in survival because of the high mortality of wounds of the heart and mediastinal structures. They may require to be managed by rotation of an adjacent muscle flap over prosthetic material or a lattice of wire sutures placed around the adjacent rib borders. Tracheostomy and intermittent positive pressure ventilation will usually be required.

References and Further Reading

Bell, M. J. (1971). The management of shotgun wounds. *Journal of Trauma*, **11**, 522–7.

De Muth, W.E. (1971). The mechanism of shotgun wounds. *Journal of Trauma,* **11,** 219–29.

Ledgerwood, A. M. (1977). The management of shotgun wounds. *Surgical Clinics of North America,* **57** (1), 111–20.

Paradies, L.H. and Gregory, C.F. (1966). The early treatment of close range shotgun wounds to the extremities. *Journal of Bone and Joint Surgery,* **48 A,** 425–35.

Sherman, R.T. and Parish, R.A. (1963). Management of shotgun injuries. A review of 152 cases. *Journal of Trauma,* **3,** 76–86.

19
Body armour

Protection of the body against damage from hand-held weapons, or projectiles, has been used since man first developed the capability of using weapons. Regrettably he found it necessary to use his newly created weapons, not only against animals, but against his fellow man.

Body armour was first made of animal hide and wood. Later as cloth was manufactured, quilted jackets were used under the armour. Metal plates, chain mail and steel armour followed, culminating in the magnificent full suits of steel armour that characterized the peak of the armourer's art. Such armour was proof against musket balls; indeed, the armour was often tested by firing at it and dents can be seen in many suits of display armour in stately homes or museums.

Throughout history emphasis in the protection has been placed on the head and trunk, because it was realized that significant wounds of these vital areas were commonly fatal whereas extremity wounds carried a better prognosis.

By the beginning of the nineteenth century, the practice of rifling the barrel of the gun became more widespread and the development of new propellants allowed bullets to be fired at velocities of over a 1000 ft/s (300 m/s). Body armour was not very effective against these bullets and went out of fashion. The first Enfield was adopted by the British Army in 1855. It fired a heavy lead bullet of 0.55 in calibre at a velocity of 1200 ft/s (400 m/s). Before the end of the century the velocity of military rifle bullets was raised to 2500 ft/s (800 m/s).

The semistatic nature of World War I led to the development of body and head armour using modern materials and techniques. At first these were variations on the original armourer's art but towards the end of the war fairly efficient protection from bullets and fragments was obtained. All such armour was basically steel plate over a padded inner layer and was fairly heavy and cumbersome.

In World War II, little work was done on armour apart from its use in protecting air crew – the flak vest. In Korea protective body armour was first used in widespread fashion by US troops and careful studies proved its value in protection against low velocity fragments. In Britain

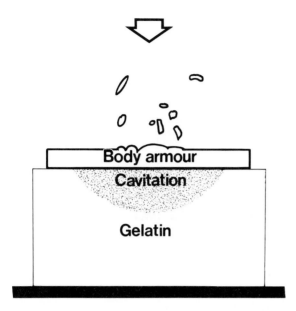

Fig. 19.1 Diagrammatic representation of an experiment in which steel armour plate rested on a gelatin simulant. The armour stopped a bullet but a small area of cavitation is seen to occur in the gelatin.

the Stores and Clothing Research Development Establishment (SCRDE) at Colchester has developed body and head armour for the British Armed Services.

Body armour can be of two main types – rigid and flexible.

Rigid armour (Fig. 19.1) works by breaking up a projectile and distributing the energy over a large area of the plate. If the plate is in direct contact with the body the shock wave can be transmitted to the underlying tissues and damage from cavitation can take place. The rigid armours are made of various metals both ferrous such as steels and nonferrous like titanium and aluminium, or of ceramics. Ceramics are extremely hard substances with a brittle front face like glass or boron carbide usually backed with a softer material which absorbs the fragments and the remaining energy. When such an armour is struck by a projectile a fracture conoid breaks out of the front face, the hardness of the front face material causes the relatively soft bullet to be eroded whilst the deformation of the backing material over the large area of the conoid base absorbs much of the energy.

Flexible armour (Fig. 19.2) works by bending under the stress and distributing the force over a large area whilst decelerating the projectile. The far side of the armour may be so distorted that it may penetrate

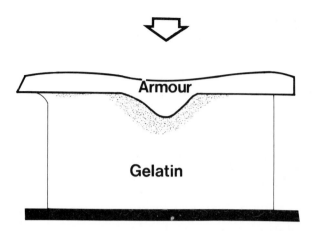

Fig. 19.2 Representation of a flexible armour which, although it stops the bullet, allows some penetration of the gelatin simulant.

the underlying tissues and minor cavitation damage can occur. For this reason both flexible and rigid armour usually carry a thick layer of padding material to help body protection (Fig. 19.3). Other new materials are tested to see if they are useful for body protection as they become

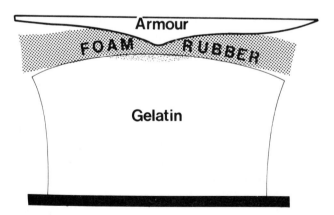

Fig. 19.3 Foam rubber or similar absorptive material, placed between the flexible armour of the rigid armour and the gelatin simulant allows the armour to stop the bullet but at the same time reduces any behind armour effects that might occur.

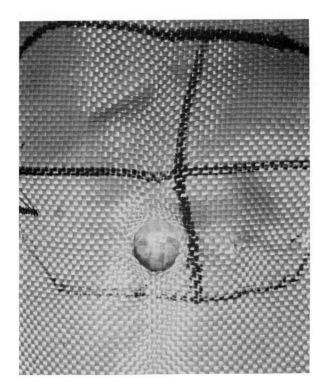

Fig. 19.4 Flexible body armour, in this case 32-ply woven Kevlar, after it has been shot at point blank range by a 9 mm automatic (7.5 g at 1150 ft/s (350 m/s)). The depression in the material is clearly shown.

available. For example when the synthetic material Kevlar became available it was first used for motor car tyres. Later it was used for many other purposes including reinforcing the hulls of yachts and, in woven form, for yacht sails. It is a very tough fibre and a number of layers of it can be put together to form a very effective, flexible and reasonably light body armour and it has the advantage that it can be made up like a waistcoat or coat. The 32-ply material is shown in Fig. 19.4 after it has been shot at point blank range by a 9 mm automatic 7.5 g at 1150 ft/s (350 m/s). The depression in the material is clearly shown. Figure 19.5 shows a bullet before firing and after impact when its squashed form was picked out of the material. The underlying bruise on the anaesthetized pig wearing such protection is shown in Fig. 19.6 and at autopsy the bruise at the subcutaneous layer is shown in Fig. 19.7. With 36-ply Kevlar there is virtually no bruise and there are no subcutaneous changes showing damage. The weight of such material, which gives excellent protection, is a problem and, therefore, a compromise may be reached

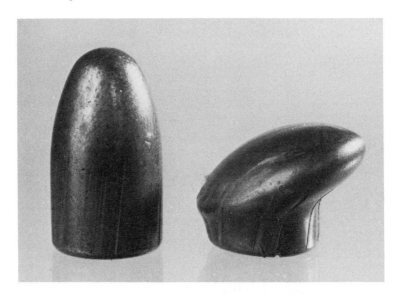

Fig. 19.5 9 mm Bullet used in the experiment to inflict damage upon the body armour shown in Fig. 19.4. On the left is the intact bullet before firing and on the right the same bullet after impact when its squashed shape was picked from the material.

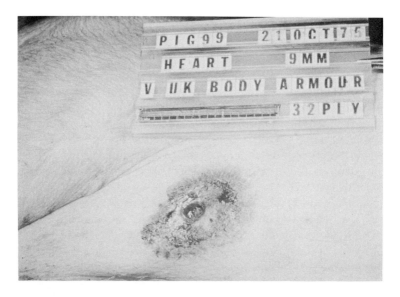

Fig. 19.6 The bruise in subcutaneous layer of an anaesthetized pig that was protected by 32-ply Kevlar flexible body armour and which was shot using a 9 mm automatic (Crown Copyright Reserved).

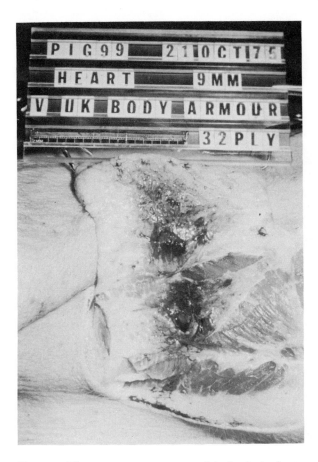

Fig. 19.7 The appearance at autopsy of the bruised subcutaneous tissues of the anaesthetized pig which was wearing flexible body armour when shot with a 9 mm automatic. (Crown Copyright Reserved)

by using 12 or 16-ply material which gives fairly good protection but is much lighter. This has been adopted by many law enforcement agencies in the USA and there are many reports of its effectiveness in protection when it has been actually struck by bullets.

Reasonably light-weight body armour is currently in use on a wide scale such as the Fragmentation Vest used by British troops in Northern Ireland (Fig. 19.8). This is made from nylon textile and will stop fragments, many hand-gun bullets and submachine guns at extended ranges. Similar protection is given by other commercial armours such as Bristol Grade 25 made of glass fibre with polyester resin (glass reinforced plastic, GRP) and used by the police in Northern Ireland.

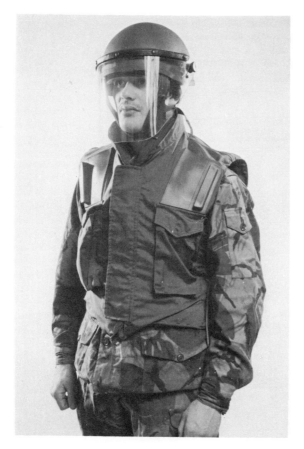

Fig. 19.8 Nylon textile fragmentation vest and helmet made of glass reinforced plastic with a polycarbonate visor, as worn by the British troops in Northern Ireland.

These materials will not protect against rifle bullets. To protect against these very high velocity missiles, a considerable weight penalty must be accepted. Armour made of steel plate or ceramic armour backed by GRP will stop the 5.56 mm and 7.62 mm rifle bullet but they all weigh about 15 kg.

Head protection is afforded, at present, by a steel helmet with a transparent visor. This is being replaced by a stronger helmet made of GRP with a polycarbonate visor as shown in Fig. 19.8. This gives good protection against crash, fragment and hand-thrown missiles, some protection against tangential hand-gun bullets but little or no protection against rifle bullets. Newer ballistic nylon materials for helmets will give even greater protection. Protection for the head against high velocity bullets is possible but the weight penalty is at least 10–12 kg.

Finally it is emphasized that protection can be offered against hand-gun bullets and fragments but against rifle bullets it is only possible to obtain adequate protection by the use of heavy materials.

General References and Further Reading

Bailey, Hamilton (ed.) (1942). *Surgery of Modern Warfare.* 2nd edn, E & S Livingstone, Edinburgh.

Beebe, G.W. and De Bakey, M.E. (1952). *Battle Casualties. Incidence, Mortality and Logistic Considerations.* Charles C Thomas, Springfield, Illinois, USA.

Cope, V.Z. (1953). *Surgery: History of the Second World War.* Medical Series, HMSO, London.

Field Surgery Pocket Book (1981). HMSO, London.

Gordon-Taylor, G. (ed.) (1947 and 1952). *British Journal of Surgery,* War Surgery Supplements, J. Wright & Sons, Bristol.

Guthrie, G.J. (1827). *On Gunshot Wounds of the Extremities.* 3rd Edn, Burgess and Hill, London.

Jolly, D.W. (1941). *Field Surgery in Total War.* Hoeber, New York.

Longmore, T. (1877). *Gunshot Injuries.* Longmans, Green & Co., London.

Melsom, M.A., Farrar, M.D. and Volkers, R.C. (1975). Battle casualties. *Annals of the Royal College of Surgeons of England,* **56,** 289–303.

NATO (1975). *Emergency War Surgery,* First revision, US Government Printing Office. Washington, DC.

Otis, G. A. (1870, 1876). *The Medical and Surgical History of the War of the Rebellion.* US Government Printing Office, Washington, DC.

Office of the Surgeon General (1955). *Surgery in World War II.* General Surgery Volumes I and II. Department of the Army, US Government Printing Office, Washington, DC.

Stevenson, W.F. (1897). *Wounds in War: the Mechanism of their Production and Treatment.* Longmans, Green & Co., London.

Trueta, J. (1939). *Treatment of War Wounds and Fractures.* Hamish Hamilton, London.

Trueta, J. (1943). *The Principles and Practice of War Surgery.* C.V. Mosby Company, St. Louis.

Watts, J. C. (1960). Military surgery: missile injuries in Cyprus. *Annals of the Royal College of Surgeons of England,* **27,** 125–43.

Whelan, T. J., Burkhalter, W. E. and Gomez, A. (1968). Management of war wounds. *Advances in Surgery,* **3,** Year Book Medical Publishers Inc., Chicago, pp. 227–349.

Wiseman, R. (1686). *Several Chirurgical Treatises.* 2nd edn, Fascimile edition of Books V, VI and VII. Kingsmead Press, Bath.

Index